Lewis & Clark

Lewis & Clark

Doctors in the Wilderness

Bruce C. Paton

Fulcrum Publishing
Golden, Colorado

Permission has been granted to reprint quotations from
The Journals of the Lewis and Clark Expedition, vols. 2–11. Gary E. Moulton, ed., University of Nebraska, Lincoln, 1997.

Library of Congress Cataloging-in-Publication Data
Paton, Bruce C.
  Lewis and Clark : doctors in the wilderness / Bruce C. Paton.
    p. cm.
  Includes bibliographical references and index.
  ISBN 1-55591-055-6 (pbk.)
  1. Lewis and Clark Expedition (1804–1806) 2. West (U.S.)—Discovery
and exploration. 3. Lewis and Clark Expedition (1804–1806)—Health
aspects. 4. Medicine—West (U.S.)—History—19th century. 5. Frontier
and pioneer life—West (U.S.) 6. Floyd, Charles, d. 1804—Health. 7. Sacagawea,
1786–1884—Health. 8. Lewis, Meriwether, 1774–1809—Health. I. Title.
F592.7.P38 2001
917.804'2—dc21

                        2001002334

Printed in the United States of America

0 9 8 7 6 5 4 3 2 1

Editorial: Daniel Forrest-Bank, Amy Timms, Alison Auch
Design: Debra B. Topping, Cyndie Chandler
Cover painting: *The Lewis and Clark Expedition,* oil on canvas, copyright © 1918
  Charles Russell. Courtesy of the Gilcrease Museum, registration #0137.2267 CT
Map: Bruce C. Paton

Fulcrum Publishing
16100 Table Mountain Parkway, Suite 300
Golden, Colorado 80403
(800) 992-2908 • (303) 277-1623
www.fulcrum-books.com

Contents

Preface

Few expeditions of any era have been scrutinized, described, discussed, and lionized as much as the Lewis and Clark exploratory trip across the continent in 1804–1806. Many wonderful books have been written, concentrating on special aspects of the journey and the journals of Lewis, Clark, Gass, Ordway, and Whitehouse have been meticulously edited. The source material available to scholars, whether serious historians or amateur enthusiasts, is enormous. The medical aspects of the trip have not received the same attention, although the work of Dr. Eldon Chuinard, *Only One Man Died,* first published in 1979 was a scholarly approach written by an orthopedic surgeon who had been a student of the expedition for many years. Since that book was written, the discipline of wilderness medicine, the study of medical care in remote and difficult situations, has developed and expanded. It is, in part, through the window of this new knowledge, that this book has been written.

The medical theories and practices of the early 1800s obviously have not changed. Some of them seem outlandish and illogical. It is hard to escape the conclusion that those who became sick on the expedition were lucky not to be made worse by the treatment they received.

There were three major medical crises: the death of Sergeant Floyd, the illness of Sacagawea, and the gunshot wound of Lewis. I have discussed the diagnoses and the treatment in all three instances, and also raised the question of what would have been the effect on the expedition if either Sacagawea or Lewis had died. Clearly, the death of Floyd had no effect on the ultimate achievements of the expedition. But that might have been different if either of the others had died.

My personal interest in the expedition arises from a lifetime enthusiasm for the outdoors, for mountains and wild places, for birds and wildlife, and for the men and women who have explored the farthest corners of our world. The Lewis and Clark expedition contains all the elements that have intrigued me for years—adventure, exploration, the discovery of new birds and animals, and personal heroism in overcoming tough and daunting environmental hazards. Other adventurers may have experienced more ghastly circumstances, fought more difficult weather, climbed higher mountains, and died seeking an unachievable grail. Perhaps the greatest success of the Lewis and Clark endeavor was that with good planning, leadership, successful diplomacy, and a good measure of luck, many of the disasters that others encountered were avoided. This success perhaps was a forerunner of future American achievements. The British, whose explorations opened up the Far North, have always prided themselves on *muddling through*, a philosophy that produced extraordinary heroism and extraordinary disaster. The Americans have prided themselves on good planning, good logistics, and adequate supplies. These principles have not always been achieved, as in the fourth journey of Frémont (1848) in the San Juan Mountains, which ended in disaster through a combination of poor leadership, poor planning, and arrogance. The comparison between the Lewis and Clark expedition and that of Frémont emphasizes the importance of leadership. Except in a few instances, the leadership of Lewis and Clark was exemplary and a major reason for their success.

The aftermath of the expedition is frustrating and sad. The route they pioneered did not turn out to be the gate to the West that President Jefferson had hoped. It took many years before the journals were published, by which time much of the critical information in them was already known. The later life histories of those who participated varied from tragic to heroic. The glue that held the men together during the trip dissolved as soon as they reached St. Louis, and Lewis died within a few years under sad and sordid circumstances. None of this, however, detracts from the glamour of the achievement, which has intrigued and inspired every generation since 1806 and will continue to excite generations to come.

A book of this sort inevitably bears the imprint of many opinions. I have sought medical advice from many friends who are more expert than I in deciphering from the scanty evidence in the journals the nature of the illnesses suffered by the members of the expedition. Those who were always helpful were Dr. Ben Eiseman, Dr. Kenneth Hovland, Dr. Dale Leichty, Dr. Stuart Schneck, Dr. William Silen, and Dr. Roger Wotkyns. In addition, I had numerous conversations with others who filled me with ideas. My editors at Fulcrum Publishing were always encouraging and sources of ideas. But, above all, I must thank my wife, Pat, for tolerating my seclusion and long silences and being a source of endless support.

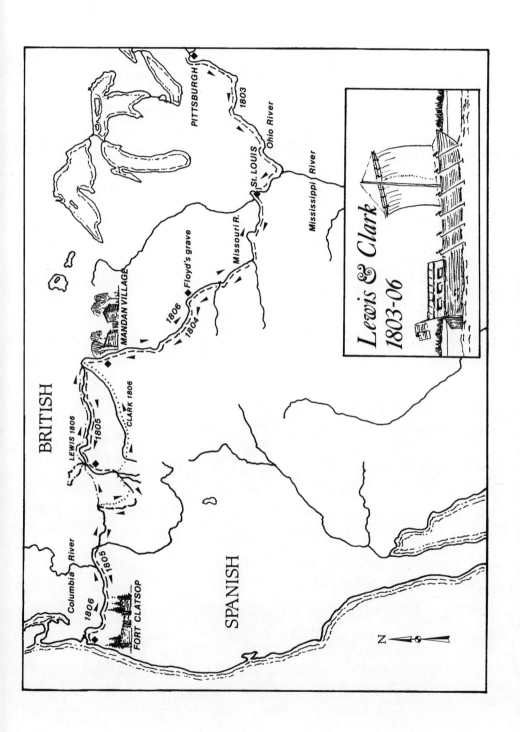

Lewis & Clark
1803-06

BRITISH

SPANISH

PITTSBURGH

1803

Ohio River

St. LOUIS

Mississippi River

Missouri R.

Floyd's grave

1806

1804

MANDAN VILLAGE

LEWIS 1806

1805

CLARK 1806

Columbia River

1805

1806

FORT CLATSOP

N

ONE

Setting the Scene

Eight men, dressed in elk-skin clothes and fur hats, strained against the current to push their long, high-prowed canoe upstream. Their skin was burned by the sun and wind to a dark mahogany, and their beards were long and thick. They spoke in rough, guttural French, salting their words with oaths and outbursts of song. The canoe was filled with bundles of beaver pelts, bound in buffalo hides: each bundle 100 pounds, a load that one man could carry over a portage. The Indians with whom the trappers had been trading beaver, buffalo, marten, and wolf skins were the Frenchmen's friends, so they did not fear sudden attack. They still had many miles to paddle and more than eighty portages to cross before reaching the warehouse of the North West Company in Montreal. That evening, as they sat around the flickering campfire, puffing on their pipes, they hoped the furs in the canoe would fetch good prices. The French Canadians had a monopoly on the trade along the upper Mississippi, and the Indians relied on the European traders for guns and ammunition, whiskey, beads, axes, blankets, and other goods. During the past few years finding beaver had become more and more difficult, but trading in beaver pelts would continue to be profitable—as long as the beavers lasted.

The driving forces behind politics and society were the same in 1800 as now—business and money. When the early Americans moved west over the Appalachians they were primarily interested in land. But as they turned their eyes beyond the Mississippi to the vast unexplored plains and mountains, they did not yet dream of gold rushes, they dreamed of furs. The French Canadians and the British had been exploring the western plains and the upper reaches of the Mississippi for many years, their long canoes returning north, laden with rich pelts, and they were always looking for new frontiers. The Americans wanted a larger piece of the action.

Expanding the fur trade was only part of the dream. For centuries explorers had been seeking a route from the Atlantic to the Pacific that would be a quicker way from Europe to the riches and markets of the Far East than the long hauls around the Cape Horn or the Cape of Good Hope. These were perilous trips that took months, even years, to finish. The English wanted to win the race to the spices, jewels, and silks of China and India. The Spanish were not as interested in the Northwest Passage because they had already found gold in Central and South America and had established trade with the Spice Islands of the East by a route around the Cape of Good Hope. The French had sought out land and trade along the valley of the Saint Lawrence River.

When the first explorers from Europe came to North America they did not have the faintest idea of the size or shape of the continent. Once the great powers, Spain, England, and France, recognized that it was a huge land mass obstructing their way west, many expeditions were sent to probe the continent, driven by trade, religion, and a desire for land. From the first the Spanish were frantic to find gold, and, finding it, they destroyed civilizations to keep it. The French soon found that the land northeast of the Great Lakes did not have gold, at least not the glittery kind they could hold in their hands. They found other gold, the soft furry kind that could be converted in the markets of the world into the hard glittery kind. And both the French and the Spanish were accompanied by priests who wanted to convert the savages to Christianity.

As soon as the great navigators of Europe recognized the land barrier between the Atlantic and the Pacific they began to think of ways to get around the continent and reach the East. There were only two maritime choices, go north or go south. The dream of a Northwest Passage was wrapped in a veil of theories, conjecture, and stories truthful and fictitious. Magellan showed that the southern route was possible, if difficult. What would the route around the north be like? Over the following years the answer came loud and strong—impossible. The attempts to find a route were heroic and frequently disastrous. But John Davis could say in 1585 that the Northwest Passage was "a matter nothing doubtful, but at any tyme almost to be passed, the sea navigable, void of use, the air tolerable and the waters very deep." He was correct on most counts except the "sea navigable." It would be more than three hundred years before Roald Amundsen took three years to squeeze his way between the icebergs and show that there was an open passage, but only if weather and the shifting ice permitted.

From the sixteenth to the beginning of the nineteenth centuries the waves of discovery waxed and waned depending on wars in Europe, treaties that meant little or nothing, relations with the Indians, and the efforts of individuals of amazing courage and energy. The French, working west from the Saint Lawrence River explored and controlled the fur trade in the lower part of Canada, out beyond the Great Lakes, and down to the upper part of the Mississippi. The Spanish established their sphere of influence in the Southwest and, for a long time, were happy with the status quo. The British based their fur trade on the Hudson Bay, and, as opposed to the French who sent their voyageurs throughout the length of the land, they built palisaded trading posts and waited for the Indians to bring their furs to them.

No exploration was more important as a precursor to the Lewis and Clark expedition than that of Louis Jolliet and Father Jacques Marquette in 1673. In 1671 the French government issued one of those statements, so typical of big colonial powers, that was both naïve and arrogant. Louis XIV, the King of France, proclaimed possession of all the lands from Montréal to the "South Sea covering the utmost extent and range possible." To further this claim Jolliet, a trader, Father Marquette, and five voyageurs canoed down the Fox River and portaged over to the Wisconsin. They traveled downstream into the Mississippi for hundreds of miles before encountering any Indians and finally ended up, far south, at the mouth of the Arkansas River, still a ten-day journey from the sea. Afraid of the Spanish, Jolliet and his men turned north for Canada. On both the downstream and the upstream journey they passed the mouth of a large river coming in from the northwest. The implications did not escape them as the Indians told them that the river led to the western ocean. How many miles away, how many portages, and how many mountains to cross they did not know. But the seed had been planted that this might be the secret to the ocean of the west. Eight years later René-Robert, Cavalier de La Salle, launched an expedition down the Illinois River to enter the Mississippi and, in April 1682, emerged into the Gulf of Mexico. He mustered a parade, and standing with his forty men he declared that France had taken possession of the Mississippi River, its tributaries, and all of the country watered by them. An immodest claim, but one that he surely believed, and one that established France's claim to a huge swath of land that eventually became the Louisiana Purchase. No one recorded what the Indians thought about it.

The size and length of the Mississippi could now be measured, but traders still had not embarked upon the mysterious river entering from the northwest, the Pettikanoui as the Indians called it. It was, of course, not the only large river coming from the West. The Osage, Kansas, and Platte rivers, all big rivers, could just as easily have been the key to the western ocean. Which of the Indian tales was to be trusted?

Explorers continued to venture westward. In 1712 Etienne Veniard de Bourgmont, a French soldier and trader, joined a group of Missouri Indians as they returned home after a war. Not content just to travel on the Missouri River and return home, he lived with the Indians for several years and journeyed 600 miles up the Missouri as far as the Platte River. Others followed, trying to make treaties with the Plains Indians, who had by now acquired horses from the Spanish, frequently by means more foul than fair, thereby increasing both their mobility and power. The French were not successful in making treaties because there was no good reason for the Indians, now the lords of the plains, to bother about a small group of strange foreigners with outrageous claims to sovereignty.

Contact with the Mandans, the nation that would be so important to Lewis and Clark, was eventually made by an extraordinary family of explorers, the Vérendryes, a father and two sons who would change the map and open the West. In April 1742 Sieur de la Vérendrye, a French Canadian, sent his sons, Le Chevalier and Francois, south across the plains from Fort La Reine on the Assiniboine River until they reached the Missouri River and the mud villages of the Mandans. While they lived with the Mandans and heard the native myths and stories, the Vérendryes concluded that the Missouri flowed from mountains separating the plains from the Pacific Ocean. They traveled farther downstream until they reached a village of the Arikaras, where they were astounded to find a chief who spoke fluent Spanish and to learn that other Frenchmen lived a few days' journey away.

For the next century French fur traders pushed their way west, river by river, lake by lake, always seeking better hunting grounds and richer furs. Most of the exploration for furs was around and to the west of the Great Lakes. But the full length of the Mississippi and the upper branches of the Missouri down to the Mandan villages, near what is now Bismarck, North Dakota, also became well known to the voyageurs.

If the continent was a physical barrier between the Atlantic and the Pacific oceans, the Mississippi River represented a psychological and political barrier between what was then the Northwest of the United States and the open, unexplored country west of the great river, then owned by France and Spain. Because the route to the Pacific was open around Cape Horn, but slow and hazardous, and the northern route was closed by walls of ice, traders and governments alike reasoned that perhaps it would be possible to find a land route or, better still, a water route, across the continent. Such a route would open trade, not only within the continent, but to the lucrative markets of China.

Priests provided many of the first accounts of the western land

and its people. The *coureurs de bois*, the hardy fur trappers who lived with and learned from the Indians, were mostly illiterate, but the priests wrote detailed reports and brought back rumors of great rivers in the West "beyond the setting sun" that led to lakes "where the water could not be drunk." The stories contained a grain of truth, but no one knew where the Indians got the stories. No Indians living along the Mississippi in the eighteenth century could ever have been to the Pacific. But perhaps, over centuries of oral history, the word had been passed from Indians on the West Coast to Indians in the Rocky Mountains, who then told it to the painted warriors of the plains and, eventually, the stories were recited around campfires along the Mississippi. It was just the old party game of sending a message from one guest to another and then listening to the final garbled version.

While the natives had their own accounts of what the landscape offered, the geographers of the day, sitting in their libraries in London and Washington, had only flimsy factual information upon which to base their ideas and draw their maps. And some of their beliefs were, in retrospect, not only wrong but distinctly weird— stories of giant volcanoes and mountains of salt, of a central lake from which rivers flowed to the oceans, or a high land mass as the source of rivers running north, south, east, and west. There were rumors of cities of gold occupied by civilized people, lost tribes of Welshmen or Jews wandering the interior west, and mammoths still roaming the plains. Perhaps the most influential and deceptive misconception was that the continent was symmetrical, with a rim of relatively low mountains in the East, a great plain in the middle and a similar rim of mountains, rivers, and plains leading to the great western sea. This idea, perhaps more than any other, convinced President Jefferson that the journey to the ocean was not only feasible but, perhaps, relatively simple. He believed that it would be possible for a small expedition to travel to the source of the Missouri River in the Rocky Mountains, carry their canoes and equipment over an easy portage to the upper reaches of the another river flowing west, and glide down to the Pacific Ocean. How did he come to this hope?

Jefferson may have been the most well-read man in the country, with an extensive library and a voracious appetite for information. He was familiar with the maps of the day and with the stories of exploration. From his youth he had been imbued with the idea of crossing the country to the Pacific. Many of Jefferson's role models, including his father, harbored goals of heading west. When Jefferson was a boy, his teacher, The Reverend James Maury, had been party to a plan in 1750 to follow the Missouri to its source and find the river that led to the western ocean. Likewise, Jefferson's father had been an investor in the Loyal Land Company that possessed extensive properties west of the Appalachians.

However, as Jefferson's political career blossomed in the latter half of the eighteenth century, territorial battles, Indian wars, and the Revolutionary War inhibited all thoughts of finding a route to the ocean. When peace came and the United States gained sovereignty over all the land east of the Mississippi, there were at least four U.S. attempts to find a route to the ocean beyond the setting sun. Jefferson was the inspiration for three of them.

In 1783 General George Rogers Clark, a hero of the Revolutionary War and elder brother to William Clark, a hero of this story, was invited by Jefferson to lead an expedition west from the Mississippi. George Clark wanted to lead a large party, but Jefferson, who was then a congressional representative from Virginia, thought that a small, unwarlike party would be better. Clark declined the offer and the plan came to naught.

While Jefferson was the Minister to France (1784–1789) he met John Ledyard, who would now be called either a soldier of fortune or a lunatic adventurer. An American from Connecticut, Ledyard had sailed under the flag of Captain James Cook in 1776 as a Corporal in the Royal Marines and had been present during the scuffle in which Cook was killed. Returning to Europe in 1785, Ledyard looked for further adventures. He conceived the idea of going around the world, mostly on foot. He obtained some support from Sir Joseph Banks in London, the doyen of exploration sponsors and a major supporter of Captain Cook. His plan had been to cross Russia, sail to the northwest coast of America, then cross the continent from west to east, on foot, accompanied by two dogs. Astonishingly, Jefferson supported Ledyard's idea, and the soon-to-be President's approval can only be explained as total, unavoidable ignorance of the geographic circumstances. Even if Ledyard had been able to reach America, the best he could have done would have been to land at Sitka, then a Russian trading post, where the impossibility of his plan would have been brought home to him. As it was, the Empress Catherine the Great had him returned to St. Petersburg and shipped out of the country before he even set sail. He died later on an expedition to the Niger River.

In 1790 another abortive attempt to organize an expedition was made by Major General Henry Knox, Secretary of War. He devised a plan for exploring the Missouri River to its source, and to search for connections between the Missouri and a river running into the Gulf of Mexico. The group, consisting of an officer and four or five "hardy Indians," would not take any written orders with them, presumably so that their intent could not be discovered if they were captured by the Spanish. A letter finally went from Knox to Lieutenant John Armstrong, the man chosen to lead the assignment. The whole idea eventually fizzled out. Armstrong started out but got nowhere. He could not find the "hardy Indians" who would be loyal and realized that he could not deceive the Spanish authorities into thinking he was a simple trader.

The American Philosophical Society, with which Jefferson was involved, organized another expedition in 1793, but that also failed. André Michaux, a French botanist who was living in the United States, was engaged to explore the Missouri and find a possible water route to the Pacific. Money was raised from members of the Society, including George Washington. No success was achieved. Michaux was in the pay of France and was soon recalled to Washington at Jefferson's urging.

Meanwhile, in 1793, Alexander Mackenzie, a hardened and experienced Scot attached to the North West Company, canoed and walked his way across the Rockies to the Pacific. He was accompanied by three associates, four voyageurs, and two Indians.

His successful transcontinental voyage demonstrated that it was possible to reach the Pacific through the Rockies. Although the route he followed was impracticable for trade, it had one attractive feature: a portage of only 800 paces across the continental divide between the Peace River running east and the Fraser River running west.

Alexander Mackenzie had spent years in the Far North and showed what it would take to succeed. On his return to London he published an account of his journey, which eventually reached Jefferson. Mackenzie's book must have influenced Jefferson's thoughts about the geography of the country, through which Lewis and Clark would eventually have to travel, especially the concept of a simple portage across the divide.

In order to know the distance from the Mississippi River to the Pacific Ocean it was obviously necessary to know more about the geography of the West Coast. The Spanish had explored the West Coast slowly and cautiously, gradually establishing missions and colonies. Every year they sent a galleon from Spain or the Philippines to resupply these small toeholds on the continent. The Spanish were not alone in wondering what the coast offered in the way of inhabitable land and riches. Sir Francis Drake, in 1579, had sailed north beyond San Francisco Bay where he landed and spent several weeks repairing his ships and becoming acquainted with the Indians. Further exploration was slow. The distances from Europe were immense, and the time taken to make any voyage involved years of planning and travel.

In the early years of the eighteenth century Peter the Great sent Vitus Bering on two expeditions along the Aleutian Peninsula, and east along the southern coast of Alaska beyond the mouth of the Copper River. Bering died before he could return to Russia, but the scorbutic survivors who finally reached home with their teeth falling out and their limbs covered with hemorrhagic sores, brought with them blankets and clothes made from the most valuable furs in the world, the pelts of sea otters and arctic foxes. In the next twenty years Russian traders, the *promyshleniki*, killed most of the Aleuts and slaughtered the otters almost to extinction.

In the last quarter of the eighteenth century the Spanish ventured farther north than they had ever dared to go, spurred on by the knowledge that the Russians were drifting down from the North. In 1775 Bruno de Hezeta sailed as far north as Nootka Sound on Vancouver Island and, on his return, passed the entrance of a large river but did not explore it. Had he done so, who knows what we would now call the Columbia River.

In the same week that the Declaration of Independence was signed in Philadelphia, the *Resolution,* a 562-ton ex-collier under the command of Captain James Cook, slipped its moorings in Plymouth and headed into the English Channel, bound for Tahiti. Cook sailed to the South Seas, making the first sightings of the Hawaiian Islands, then turned north, searching once more for the elusive Northwest Passage. The ship sailed up the Alaskan coast, turned west to present-day Anchorage, then headed down along and around the Aleutian Peninsula, before venturing northward through the Bering Strait, only to be turned back by a wall of ice. There was no Northwest Passage this way. Cook sailed south again and returned to the Hawaiian Islands where he met his death under the war clubs of the natives. By the end of this voyage the shape and conformation of the Alaskan coast had been delineated. All that remained was to explore the ins and outs of the coast and find the mouths of the rivers that the geographers had for years speculated emptied into the Pacific.

In 1792 Captain Robert Gray, an American, sailed into the huge mouth of the river that he named the Columbia, after his ship. Not long after that, Captain George Vancouver, leading a British naval expedition, sent a junior officer, Lieutenant William Broughton, up the Columbia for more than 100 miles until the rapids—which would also be a source of trouble to Lewis and Clark—stopped further progress. The explorers pinpointed the exact longitude and latitude of the mouth of the Columbia, and as a result, geographers could then measure the exact distance between St. Louis and the West Coast. They could only guess what lay between.

By the time Thomas Jefferson became President of the United States he hoped that not only could furs trapped in the West be brought back quickly to the eastern United States through the mountains and down the rivers, but that those caught on the West Coast could be shipped directly to the markets of Canton and Shanghai. Furs trapped west of the Great Lakes sometimes took two years to reach Montreal. There had to be a shorter and more profitable route that would also take the trade away from the British.

The time was ripe for Jefferson to fulfill his hopes, and his election to the presidency in 1800 made this possible. Soon after moving into the half-built White House he invited a young officer, Meriwether Lewis, well known to Jefferson through family connections, to become his Secretary. There are strong suggestions that the appointment was more than a gesture toward a family friend, and that Jefferson had already decided Lewis would head the expedition to the West Coast that he had planned for some years.

Despite the timing, there was a major difficulty in planning an expedition to penetrate the country west of the Mississippi: France owned the land. Originally a French claim, the land was ceded to Spain in 1762, and in 1800, by a secret treaty, returned to the French. Fortunately for Jefferson and America, Napoleon embarked on an ill-fated campaign. He sent an army of about forty-six thousand men to Santo Domingo, now Haiti, to stop a slave uprising. The French Army was decimated by yellow fever and could not sustain the campaign. Napoleon subsequently wanted to extract himself from an untenable situation and, as war was again looming on the horizon in Europe, decided to sell Louisiana to the Americans. Jefferson had sent plenipotentiaries to Paris hoping, perhaps, to buy New Orleans or come to some arrangement that would permit free trade through the port. To the surprise of the Americans and the delight of Jefferson, who did not know about the details of the deal until it had been consummated, Napoleon sold all the French possessions west of the Mississippi to the Americans for $15 million. (This purchase is often referred to as being dirt cheap; but in year-2001 dollars it probably cost about $300 million—still a great bargain.) The outlook for an expedition changed overnight. No longer would the men be sneaking through someone else's territory. They would be marching on American soil.

Before the Louisiana Purchase Jefferson had already started to lay the foundations for an expedition. He knew that, for various reasons, Congress would never appropriate money for an expedition that had to go through Spanish or French territory. On January 18, 1803, Jefferson sent a politically ingenious, confidential message to Congress. He started by writing about the Indians and their gradual move westward as their land was sold to Americans. Jefferson wanted the Indians to turn from hunting to agriculture. Next he emphasized that he wanted to increase the number of trading houses in the Indian territories "and place within their reach those things which will contribute more to their domestic comfort." All this sounded very reasonable. He then moved from discussing Indians in general to specifically addressing the tribes along the Missouri River and how they furnished great supplies of "furs and peltry to the trade of another nation through an infinite number of portages and lakes, shut up by ice through a long season." He was, of course, referring to the British fur trade routes along the northern Mississippi and the Missouri that extended north to Montreal. The route for that trade, he explained, could never be as good as a more southerly route along the Missouri that could join with a river route to the western ocean "possibly with a single portage." He proposed an expedition with ten or twelve chosen men, led by an adept officer, to explore western Indian country and obtain admission for traders. The hook was at the end of the message: "The appropriation of two thousand five hundred dollars for the purpose of extending the external commerce of the U.S."

Jefferson got his money and then, deceptively, started spreading the information that the expedition would be up the Mississippi, not the Missouri. He was anxious that the true intent of the expedition, to explore a route to the Pacific Ocean, not become known to the Spanish and French. Not everyone was deceived. As soon as the Congress agreed to give the money the wheels of preparation began to roll. Jefferson gave Meriwether Lewis instructions to get started, gather the supplies, and muster the men.

Meriwether Lewis, born in Albermarle County in Virginia in 1774, was the son of William Lewis, who died during the Revolutionary War, not from a wound, but while returning to his unit. While crossing a river his horse was swept away and drowned. William Lewis struggled home, cold and wet, and caught pneumonia from which he died. Meriwether's mother, whose maiden name was Lucy Meriwether, soon married again to Captain John Marks. Lucy Lewis Marks, a singularly energetic and capable woman, was a powerful influence in the life of the young Meriwether. She was a well-known figure in the county and took her young son with her while she visited sick neighbors and servants. It was during these excursions that Meriwether probably learned much about herbs and simples, the basis for medicines of the day, and began to recognize the patterns of disease—fevers, infections and abscesses, lacerations and sprains.

When Meriwether was nine he moved with his family to Georgia where a new colony was developing. Those were exciting, formative years for the young boy: hunting, riding horses, and studying birds and animals. He learned to love the wildness of the country and became fearless in exploring the forests on his own. After a few years in Georgia, Meriwether was sent back to Virginia to receive a more formal education, although he never attended a school as we now know them. During the next few years he received instruction from various teachers and, at the same time, learned the management of the large estate he had inherited from his father. He maintained a loving relationship with his mother by frequent letters and repeatedly wrote that he wanted to return to Georgia. He did eventually return to Georgia to organize the return of his mother, servants, and family back to Virginia. This experience, too, must have strengthened his organizational skills. By the age of eighteen he was on his own and entered into the life of a wealthy young Virginian: racing horses, attending parties, overseeing the estate's slaves, and selling tobacco and produce.

In 1792, when Lewis heard about the American Philosophical Society's proposed expedition, he approached Jefferson with the hope of being chosen to lead the adventure. It was probably just as well that Michaux was sent. Lewis was not adequately experienced, the Louisiana Purchase had not been made, Jefferson was not President and the proposed group was too small to succeed.

The Whiskey Rebellion of 1794 gave Lewis the chance to join the Army. The farmers and settlers of the West had refused to pay a new tax on whiskey. Whiskey, after all, was not only something to drink, its production was a livelihood and a way of life. The war turned out to be less than a war. The rebels did not want to get into a pitched battle, and the initial retribution that was brought down on them was less than fair. In addition, the Army was neither well disciplined nor well supplied. The lower ranks had inadequate food and clothing, while the officers lived in private homes. Lewis, who enlisted as a private, was privileged, because of his family background, to have better treatment. When he became an officer he was even happier with military life, but he also came to face-to-face with the realities of being an officer.

As an officer, Lewis was responsible for the lives, discipline, and health of his men. The officers in the Army of that time often had to act as doctors. The men were frequently sick with dysentery or malaria and, in addition, poor discipline led to ferocious floggings for simple offenses. Lewis must have had to deal with injuries and illnesses he had never previously encountered. When the war ended Lewis prolonged his service by enlisting full-time as an ensign in the Army. He remained on the frontier, mostly in what is now Ohio, gaining experience in wilderness travel, in dealing with the Indians, and in military leadership. Unknowingly, he was training for what lay ahead.

Lewis' military service was not without rough spots. He was fond of drink, and once, while drunk, made ungentlemanly remarks to another officer whom he challenged to a duel. Dueling was illegal in the Army, so Lewis was tried but acquitted of the charges. His next assignment was to an elite unit of sharpshooters in which his commanding officer was William Clark. Lewis served under Clark for only six months, but, in that short time, a strong bond of confidence developed between them that would later blossom into one of the great comradeships of history.

William Clark was four years older than Lewis. He had moved from Virginia, where he was born, to Kentucky when he was a teenager. As a young man he too experienced life on the frontier which, at that time, extended no farther than the western Appalachians. He joined the Army in 1792 and fought in the campaign against the Indians under General Anthony Wayne (1794). Clark had considerably more exposure to fighting than did Lewis and was a more outgoing character, finding it easy to get along with his men. He was also an admirer of the Indians. He left the Army in 1796 with the rank of Captain and kept in touch with Lewis intermittently over the next few years. But he must have been surprised to receive a letter from the Secretary to the President, dated June 19, 1803. The letter started off with some business concerning papers belonging to George Rogers Clark, but Lewis soon urged William to keep the contents of the letter secret before launching into an account of the expedition and what the voyage hoped to achieve. Only toward the end of the letter did Lewis broach the possibility that Clark might come with him. "If, therefore, there is anything under these circumstances, in this enterprise, which

---

Historians have speculated why Jefferson chose Meriwether Lewis to lead the Corps of Discovery. Did Jefferson appoint Lewis as his Secretary with the expedition to the West in mind? Donald Jackson, a Lewis and Clark historian, argued otherwise. Lewis was not only a family friend. He had served in the Army during the Whiskey Rebellion and then remained in the service, although mostly in administrative positions. As a paymaster Lewis traveled from unit to unit and was very familiar with the officers serving in the Ohio Valley. Jefferson needed a secretary who knew the political loyalties of the officer corps, and Lewis had the inside information that Jefferson wanted. Jackson reasoned that the decision to appoint Lewis as the leader of the expedition came later.

---

would induce you to participate with me in its fatiegues, its dangers and its honors, believe me there is no man on earth with whom I should feel equal pleasure in sharing them as with yourself."

Clark replied: "Clarksville, July 18th, 1803. Dear Lewis: I received by yesterday's mail your letter of the 19th ulto. The contents of which I received with much pleasure. . . . I will cheerfully join you in an 'official Charrector' as mentioned in your letter and partake in the dangers, difficulties and fatigues. . . . This is an undertaking fraited with many difficulties, but, My friend I do assure you that no man lives whith whome I would prefer to undertake Such a Trip &c. as yourself, and I shall arrange my matters as well as I can against your arrival here." Without hesitation Clark agreed with the plan, except that he seemed to want a bigger group than that proposed. He started to look for men to join the expedition, and thus the Corps of Discovery was established.

TWO

Putting It Together

L ooking back over the last two centuries, during which thousands of explorations have been launched, the speedy and sometimes almost casual way in which the Lewis and Clark endeavor was put together is quite amazing. Congress appropriated funding soon after Jefferson's proposal in January 1803 and by August 31, the expedition had pushed off from Pittsburgh and was headed down the Ohio River. In those eight months Lewis not only had to decide what equipment he needed, but he also had to arrange for many of the supplies to be made. He visited the Army Arsenal at Harper's Ferry to choose weapons and construct a special collapsible boat. He begged, borrowed, and bought additional weapons, medicines, food, clothing, camping equipment, scientific instruments, tools for carpentry, and much else. On the orders of the President he also visited numerous famous authorities to refresh his scientific knowledge. And he had to choose a deputy commander— a task that he delayed until a few weeks before departure. Up to the last day Lewis was dickering over transporting the equipment to Pittsburgh, the expedition's starting place. On top of it all he had to have a boat built that would take his crew down the Ohio and much of the way up the Missouri. And, when he set off down the Ohio, he had not selected any of the soldiers who would be the mainstay of the group, soon to be named the Corps of Discovery. To our modern-day amazement, he did it all without a telephone, computer, or assistant—only a slow and unreliable postal service. The results speak for themselves.

Congress had provided a budget of $2,500 to pay for the initial expenses including, provisions, medicines, guns, ammunition, gifts for the Indians, and scientific equipment. However, they had not been as penny-pinching as it might seem. Figures kept by the U.S. government going back to 1866 indicate that one dollar then would be worth seventeen dollars now. Allowing for some guesswork, it would be reasonable to think that a dollar in 1803 might now be worth twenty dollars. Therefore, using this formula, Lewis was given the equivalent of $50,000 to spend. (The final cost of the expedition in year-2001 dollars was about $700,000.)

Lewis' first task was to visit the Army Arsenal at Harper's Ferry where he selected rifles and other weapons for the journey. The arsenal had just designed a new short rifle that was more accurate and easier to carry and load than the older, longer models. These became the hunters' favorite weapon.

Buying rifles was not Lewis' only mission at the arsenal. He wanted to build a collapsible boat to use on the upper reaches of the Missouri. (A large 55-foot keelboat, a common design used on the Mississippi and capable of carrying more then 3 tons, was to be built in Pittsburgh for the deeper sections of the river.) In the upper sections of the river it would be necessary to have a shallow-draft boat that could still carry a large load but that would not be as massive as the keelboat. Lewis designed a collapsible metal frame over which hides could be stretched to make a light, portable boat that would carry at least 1,500 pounds. He spent a lot of time, longer than he anticipated, designing the frame and having it made. This was to be his special baby. He spent so much time at the arsenal that Jefferson became concerned about more delays causing a later start for the expedition.

After spending about a month at the arsenal, Lewis went to Philadelphia to fulfill the instructions Jefferson had given him. The days spent there must have been both intense and fascinating. For a young man, only twenty-nine years old, entrusted with leading the greatest expedition into unexplored Indian territory yet planned on behalf of the new country, and given introductions to the finest minds of the age, those were heady days. Hard work by day and socializing with geniuses by night.

In addition to obtaining supplies, Jefferson instructed Lewis to prepare himself for the trip intellectually by honing some of his skills and acquiring others. Jefferson was President of the American Philosophical Society, the oldest and most distinguished scientific society in the country, so he called on his friends, the best authorities in their fields, to help prepare the young officer for the tasks ahead. Andrew Ellicott, a well-known surveyor, taught Lewis how to use a sextant and chronometer. Robert Patterson, Professor of Mathematics at the University of Pennsylvania, devised a cipher for sending secret messages back to Washington and supplied Jefferson with a whimsical and prophetic example to show its potential use, "I am at the head of the Missouri. All well. And the Indians, so far, friendly." Dr. Benjamin Smith Barton, a noted botanist, taught Lewis about the preservation of animal and botanical specimens. Dr. Caspar Wistar, Professor of Anatomy at the University of Pennsylvania, shared his knowledge about geology and fossils and also provided Lewis with the latest reports on the geography of the Mississippi and Missouri River valleys.

In order to upgrade his medical knowledge and to learn about matters concerning health and disease Lewis consulted Dr. Benjamin Rush, one of the leading physicians of the time and Jefferson's personal medical advisor. Lewis must have wondered what medical problems he might encounter, and an opportunity to meet with a physician as distinguished as Benjamin Rush must have been both intimidating and exhilarating.

Jefferson had written to Rush asking him to provide Lewis with questions about the Indians and also to give him medical advice. Benjamin Rush had been a signer of the Declaration of Independence as well as a Professor of Chemistry at the College of Philadelphia and, later, Professor of Medicine at the University of Pennsylvania. He may have been a friend of the President, but he was not always popular amongst his peers. He was contentious, opinionated, and did not take criticism well, but he was knowledgeable and had a long-standing interest in the culture and diseases of the Indians.

On March 12, 1803, Rush replied to Jefferson's request in a long letter that also included advice about a chronic bowel condition that seemed to have been troubling the President. Rush advised Jefferson to take laudanum before going to bed. If the laudanum did not work, he advised Jefferson to apply blisters to his wrists and ankles. "Such is the sympathy between the skin and the bowels, that the irritation of the blisters on the skin suspends all morbid action in the bowels." The blisters on the skin were so irritating that the unfortunate patient was likely to forget about his bowels: an ancient theory called "counter irritation." Toward the end of the letter Rush included a single sentence referring to Lewis: "I shall expect to see Mr. Lewis in Philadelphia, and shall not fail of furnishing him with a number of questions calculated to increase our knowledge of subjects connected with medicine." The President's bowels seemed to be of more interest and importance to Dr. Rush than the visit of an unknown presidential aide.

Lewis visited Rush soon after and received both medical advice and the promised questions to be researched. On June 11, 1803, Rush was able to report to President Jefferson, "I have endeavored to fulfil your wishes by furnishing Mr. Lewis with some inquiries relative to the natural history of the Indians. The enclosed letter contains a few short directions for the preservation of his health, as well as the health of the persons under his command."

Rush's knowledge of Indian diseases had not come from close contact with the tribes, but from assiduous questioning of others who passed through Philadelphia. He never let pass an opportunity to ask an experienced visitor about the culture and illnesses of the Indians. In 1774 he gave a speech to the American Philosophical Society in which he discussed the Indian practices and praised them for their use of bleeding. "To know that opening a vein in the arm, or foot, would relieve pain in the head or the side, supposes some knowledge of the animal economy, and therefore marks an advanced period in the history of medicine."

The questions Rush asked Lewis to answer were those he had been asking others for many years. In 1790 Rush asked the Chief of the Creek tribe, whom he had met, a series of questions about childbirth, children's mortality, suicide, the effects of aging on mental acuity, and sexuality. A year later Rush sent a list of eighteen similar questions to someone about to visit the Seneca Indians. In this list he added questions about exhaustion, menstruation, the weaning of children, and the prevalence of venereal disease. Rush posed similar questions to Lewis in three categories: physical history and medicine, morals, and religion—most of which he had asked others before, with one addition—what of Indian remedies?

1. Physical History and Medicine

1. What are the acute diseases of the Indians? Is the bilious fever attended with a black vomit?
2. Are goiter, apoplexy, palsy, epilepsy, madness, and venereal diseases known among them?
3. What is their state of life as to longevity?
4. At what age do the women begin and cease to menstruate? At what age do they marry? How long do they suckle their children?
5. What is the provision of their children after being weaned?
6. The state of the pulse as to frequency in the morning, at noon & at night—before and after eating? What is its state in childhood, adult life and old age? The number of strokes counted by the quarter of a minute by glass, and multiplied by four will give its frequency in a minute.
7. What are their remedies?
8. Are artificial discharges of blood ever used among them?
9. In what manner do they induce sweating?
10. Do they ever use voluntary fasting?
11. At what time do they rise (and have) their baths?
12. What is their diet—manner of cooking & times of eating among the Indians?
13. How do they preserve their food?

2. Morals
1. What are their vices?
2. Is suicide common among them?—ever from love?
3. Do they employ any substitute for ardent spirits to promote intoxication?
4. Is murder common among them, & do they punish it with death?

3. Religion
1. What affinity (is there) between their religious ceremonies & those of the Jews?
2. Do they use animal sacrifices in their worship?
3. What are the principal objects of their worship?
4. How do they dispose of their dead, and with what ceremonies do they inter them?

These questions show Rush's wide-ranging interests. Not only was he inquisitive about specific diseases, but he also wanted to learn about basic physiological and social facts among Native Americans including pulse rates, menstruation, and child rearing. How much better informed we would be if he had explained his thinking behind the questions. Why did he want to know an Indian's pulse rate *after* meals? Feeling the pulse is an important part of physical assessment. Doctors in the nineteenth century were concerned not only with the rate but the strength and fullness, the regularity and rhythm. The same issues concern doctors today. It is interesting that Rush felt he had to explain how to count the pulse rate per minute. The method he described is the same one used today by the nurse in your doctor's office.

Unfortunately, Lewis' journals do not mention any study of the pulse rates among Native Americans. If Lewis had checked the pulse rates of the Indians, who were generally quite athletic, he would probably have found that they had lower resting rates than Rush was used to measuring in the more sedentary residents of Philadelphia. The pulse rate, both at rest and during exercise, is related to a person's state of physical fitness. The Indians, being very active, would most likely have had slow resting pulse rates, perhaps as low as 55 to 60 beats per minute. In contrast, the more sedentary burghers of Philadelphia could have had resting pulse rates of around 70 beats per minute. Rush's conclusion would have, perhaps, been that there was some physiologic difference between the races.

It is not surprising that Rush also inquired about "artificial discharges of blood," considering his interest in bleeding as an important, even essential, treatment for many diseases. Some Indians used scarification, the abrasion of skin over a painful area, but it wasn't until coming in contact with European medicine that most North American Indian tribes began bleeding their sick. Central and South American tribes, such as the Aztecs, did bleed to relieve illness and cut the scalp to cure headaches. Reports written at the time of the Lewis and Clark expedition indicate that while some Indians used bleeding, they never bled to the point of faintness, as was frequently the custom of the day among white doctors.

Benjamin Rush, the advising physician to the Lewis and Clark expedition, was a man with many interests. He started the original post office, organized the first tax-free schools for poor children, encouraged education for women, and helped to establish American psychiatry and cures for mental diseases. He was one of the founders of the College of Physicians and promoted the Philadelphia Dispensary that treated eight thousand poor people in its first five years. Rush was a vociferous citizen who opposed public punishment and executions. He warned that by moving the U.S. capital from Philadelphia to Washington the legislators would "have mosquitoes your sentinels by night and bilious fevers your companions every summer and fall, and pleurisy every spring."

In addition, Rush wanted to know whether certain diseases such as goiter, apoplexy, epilepsy, and madness were known among the Indians. Goiter, an enlargement of the thyroid gland at the base of the neck is due to iodine deficiency. The thyroid needs iodine to produce the hormones that control the metabolism of the body. In the middle of large continents such as Asia, Africa, and America, far from an ocean, there is a lack of iodine in the water, and even in the fish in the rivers. As a result, the dietary intake of iodine is less than needed for health, and the thyroid enlarges as it attempts to make use of the limited iodine available. Women, who require more iodine than men, are still seen in some parts of the world with huge thyroids hanging like a pair of oranges at the base of the neck, filling up the space between chin and chest. Rush did not know the cause of goiter, as no one was aware of the thyroid gland's function in 1803, let alone its relationship to iodine. Many years would pass before that information became available. Yet, perhaps he knew that large thyroid glands were common in Indians, and, once more, he wanted to understand the differences between Indians in the East and those in the West.

Years after the Lewis and Clark expedition Rush became intensely interested in the treatment of mental disease. Apoplexy, epilepsy, and madness were all considered to be manifestations of mental disease, which was thought of as a continuing fever. Most patients with mental problems were incarcerated in terrible institutions that discredited the name "hospital." Rush cared for his own son in such an institution for twenty-seven years. The patients were chained in cold cells and treated with a severity not meted out to the horses in the streets. As Rush became older his thoughts changed, and he began to see that this "treatment" was not only brutal, but also ineffective. Rush has since become known as one of the fathers of psychiatry, and it is clear from the questions he posed to Lewis that he was already wondering about the workings of the mind as well as the body.

The question about venereal disease is strange considering Rush's knowledge of the Indians. Rush must have known that venereal diseases had been rampant among the Indians and in the Army for many years. It was an accepted feature of military life. He was well aware of this but, perhaps, was interested in finding how far the diseases had spread and how prevalent they were. Even in 1803 there was discussion about the origins of syphilis. Had it been introduced from Europe or was it indigenous to the Americas? Rush, who believed that venereal disease had been introduced and was not indigenous, may have wondered if it was unknown in a population isolated from previous contact with Europeans. If so, the belief that syphilis had been introduced would gain strength. There were very few Indian nations that had not had some contact with Europeans, even if only indirectly. The chances of finding a totally isolated community were slim. Finding an Indian cure would obviously have been important.

Rush was also curious about menstruation. We now know that cultural and ethnic differences do not affect physiologic functions such as menstruation. But, back then, it was reasonable that Rush might wonder about possible differences. If people were of a different color and had different habits, diet, diseases, and longevity, might not their body functions be different? And what about their vices? One person's vice may be another's normal behavior. Rush did not necessarily want to impose his values on the Indians, but he would certainly have regarded sexual license, murder, robbery, and drunkenness as vices.

As far as we know, Rush never received formal answers to his questions after the expedition returned home. Had Rush lived long enough—he died in 1813—he would have found many of the questions answered inferentially in the published journals, even the question concerning Jewish rituals. The journals, with the exception of Sergeant Patrick Gass's, were not published until after Rush died, but he must surely have inquired about the findings of the expedition after they returned.

In addition to posing questions, Rush also provided Lewis with medical advice. Rush couched his advice about maintaining health in ten simple statements.

1. Wear flannel next to the skin, especially in winter.

2. Always take a little raw spirits after being very wet or much fatigued; and as little as possible at any other time.

3. When you feel the least indisposition, fast and rest; and dilute [your] drinks for a few hours, take a sweat, and if costive [constipated] take a purge of two pills every four hours until the bowels operate freely.

4. Unusual costiveness is often a sign of approaching disease. When you feel it, take one or two of the opening pills.

5. Where salt cannot be had with your meat, steep it a day or two in common lye.

6. In difficult and laborious enterprises or marches, eating sparingly will enable you to bear them with less fatigue and more safety to your health.

7. Wash [your] feet with spirit when chilled and every morning with cold water.

8. [Drink] molasses or sugar with water with victuals and for drink with meals.

9. Wear shoes without heels.

10. Lie down when fatigued.

This advice was simple, harmless, often inappropriate, and, in some respects, ridiculous. Some of the advice was not only impracticable but bore no relation to the circumstances of the journey. Rush was a city dweller who had never experienced prolonged travel in wild and unknown places, and his advice reflects this lack of experience and understanding. To advise washing the feet with cold water every morning to a group that was about to haul heavy boats up one of the greatest rivers in the continent, makes one wonder how well he understood the full meaning of the journey. Lewis could have received better advice from his mother, his first medical teacher.

Although Rush provided these simple suggestions, there is no indication in Rush's collected letters, or in Lewis' journal, that Rush provided either written or verbal information about his favorite therapeutic methods. During the days Lewis spent with Rush they must have discussed the indications and methods for bleeding. Rush had a near obsession with bleeding as a cure for all ills, and it is amazing that this was not mentioned in the list of remedies. Bleeding was such a common treatment for illness that every member of the expedition must have been bled at some time in his life. Lewis certainly expected to bleed his men, because three fine lancets for bleeding were included in his medical kit. Likewise, Rush's advice about purging, another popular method of treatment, was quite mild, although the pills Rush prescribed were far from moderate. Made from combined doses of two potent laxatives, they were not called "Rush's Thunderbolts" for nothing.

Rush based much of his advice on his experience in the Revolutionary Army. During the war he had been Medical Director of the Middle District and had witnessed the horrors of the battlefield and the military hospitals. He had the soldiers wear flannel, similar to that worn centuries before by the Roman legionnaires. The wearing of heavy flannel was believed to prevent camp infections. Malaria, which was widespread during the summer throughout the eastern United States, could immobilize an army. Rush, like most doctors of the time, believed that malaria was due to noxious emanations from the environment. Thus its name "mal-aria." "It is a well known fact," he wrote—and how often does that phrase precede something that is neither well known nor fact—"that the perspiration of the body, by attaching itself to linen and afterwards mixing with rain, is disposed to form miasmata which produces fevers." Rush believed that flannel would prevent perspiration from soaking the clothing and evaporating into the air to cause fever. Dense flannel shirts may indeed have been better than those made of thin cotton for a totally different reason. It was more difficult for the proboscis of malaria-ridden mosquitoes to pierce a thick barrier of flannel than a thin barrier of sweaty cotton.

In the nineteenth century the diagnosis of fevers was a guessing game. The cause of malaria was not understood, and the "ague," while often due to malaria, could equally be due to other causes. As Rush knew nothing about the specific causes and epidemiology of fevers the expedition might encounter, any advice he gave about treating fevers was nothing more than speculation.

Rush had many firmly held biases: some good, some bad. Heavy drinking was part of the military life, and yet he believed resolutely that strong spirits were bad and that their consumption did nothing to protect soldiers from cold or exhaustion. Rum, he wrote, "lays the foundation of fevers, fluxes and the jaundice." In spite of Rush's antipathy to liquor for soldiers, when the Corps finally left their winter quarters at Camp Dubois, near St. Louis, in April 1804 they took with them 120 gallons of whiskey that lasted until July 4, 1805.

Rush's stint in the military also influenced his standards for medical care. The morbidity and mortality that he witnessed in military hospitals was calamitous, and he described them as the "sinks of human life in the army." He had advised that soldiers who were sick would be much better off being lodged at local farms where they could get a wholesome diet rather than staying in pest-infested hospitals. And he believed that soldiers should eat a vegetarian diet rather than the three to five pounds of meat they received every day. Perhaps he did not give this advice to Lewis because he realized that it would not sit well with a group of hungry soldiers who were going to live off the land, and whose main source of food would be the animals they shot. Had he known how many buffalo, elk, and deer it would take to satisfy their appetites, he would have gasped with amazement. At one time the hunters for the expedition brought in thirty-two deer, twelve elk, and one buffalo—but this barely lasted three weeks.

After spending the first winter at the Mandan camp, Lewis wrote back to Jefferson, "Since our arrival in this place we have subsisted principally on meat with which our guns have supplied us amply, and have thus been enabled to reserve the parched meal, portable soup, and a considerable portion of pork and flour which we had intended for the more difficult parts of our voyage." A vegetarian diet was not even worth suggesting.

While Rush avoided dietary recommendations he was certainly curious about other daily habits. Why did he inquire about the bathing habits of the Indians? People did not consider showers and baths the essential part of daily life they do now. Plumbing was rudimentary, and running hot and cold water were unknown luxuries in homes. Puritanical views discouraged bathing, except in medicinal springs. Rush himself was not a great enthusiast for total immersion. When he was in his twenties he once confided to a friend that he had recently taken a shower, the first time his body had been totally washed for more than twenty years. Regardless, he asked Lewis to investigate how and why the Indians bathed.

After receiving all of these instructions Lewis still had to go shopping for the remaining supplies. Philadelphia was the ideal place. Israel Whelan, the Purveyor of Public Supplies, was Lewis' buying agent and guide. The two men must have spent many hours in warehouses along the docks or poking down narrow, cobbled streets seeking out special merchants. The expedition's shopping list included 170 different items, and many dozens of some of those items. There were mathematical and scientific instruments, clothing, arms and ammunition, camp equipment, provisions, gifts for the Indians, boats and boat hardware, and medicines and medicine chests. Many items, such as mosquito nets, were to protect the health of the men. The nets were brought for comfort and were greatly missed when they were left behind or became so tattered that they were ineffective. Lewis purchased remarkably little food, because most of it was to be acquired by bartering or hunting along the way. One hundred and fifty pounds of portable soup and quantities of dried grains that would last a long time were taken as emergency supplies. Portable soup was an obnoxious but nutritious concoction that would keep for many months. It was made from boiling cow hooves and other sources of protein and adding vegetables and allowing the mess to gel. As cow hooves are the basis for making glue, one can only imagine how the soup tasted. The British Navy had used similar portable soups during long sea voyages as emergency rations. The soup was never intended to be a part of the regular diet.

Benjamin Rush had advised Lewis about medical supplies prior to the shopping spree. He went to the apothecaries of Gillaspay and Strong with a final list that contained thirty-two different medications or applications, plus instruments and containers (see Table 1). These supplies were chosen in accordance with the three major therapeutic principles of the day: bleeding, purging with laxatives, and cleansing the gastrointestinal tract with emetics and enemas. The supplies Lewis bought, therefore, were carefully selected and reflected the medical thinking of the day. Various laxatives (jalap, calomel, rhubarb, cream of tartar, Glauber's salts, magnesia, and nutmeg) topped the list with a total of nearly five thousand doses. Rush's Bilious Pills—also called Rush's Thunderbolts—were notorious in 1803, but Lewis also took many doses of Glauber's salts, calomel, cream of tartar and jalap for the same purposes. Compared with laxatives, only a small amount of emetics, used to induce vomiting, (ipecacuan, white vitriol, and tartar) were taken, close to three hundred doses.

Gastric and intestinal disorders were an everyday occurrence in the early nineteenth century. Sanitation was poor and there was no understanding of the need for clean handling of food. Army doctors were well aware that men remained healthier if they did not have to stay for a long time in one place but could instead move their camps frequently. And it was known that latrines should be built far from a camp. The Corps was probably protected from many minor intestinal scourges by constant movement from one place to another.

The management of fever was a constant problem for the Corps, especially in the summer months. Malaria was widespread throughout the eastern states and in the Mississippi Valley. How far it had spread up the Missouri at the time of the expedition is not known, but it was becoming an established problem on the West Coast. As things turned out, the Corps remained remarkably free of serious fevers, but to take nearly three thousand doses of Peruvian bark from which quinine is extracted was a good precaution. The bark could also be used for other fevers and as a poultice for injuries, including snakebites.

TABLE 1—*Medical supplies taken on the expedition:*

15 lbs Peruvian bark	4 oz Laudanum
1/2 lb Jalap	2 lbs Basilicum ointment
1/2 lb Rhubarb	Calamine
4 oz Ipecac	Epispastric
2 lbs Cream of Tartar	Mercury ointment
2 oz Gum Camphor	Emplast
1 lb Assafoetida	1 set Pocket Instruments
1/2 lb Opium	1 set dental instruments
1/4 lb Tragacanth	1 Clyster syringe
6 lbs Glauber Salts	4 Penis syringes
2 lbs Saltpeter	3 Best Lancets
2 lbs Ferrous Sulfate	1 Tourniquet
6 oz Lead Acetate	2 oz Patent Lint
1 oz Tartar Emetic	50 doz Rush's Bilious Pills
4 oz White Vitriol	6 Tin canisters
1/2 lb Root of Columbo	3 – 8 oz Stoppered bottles
1/4 lb Sulphuric Acid	5 – 4 oz Tincture bottles
1/4 lb Wintergreen	1 Walnut chest
1/4 lb Copaiboe	1 Pine chest
1/4 lb Benzoin	2 oz Magnesia
1/4 lb Indian ink	2 oz Gum elastic
2 oz Nutmegs	2 oz Cloves
5 oz Cinnamon	

The amount of opium that Lewis packed, 8 ounces, has been cal-culated to be enough for a total of three doses a day, every day, for the duration of the expedition. This generous amount was perhaps based on a plan to leave caches of medicines and supplies along the way that could be retrieved on the return journey from the coast. Opium relieved the pain of wounds and was an excellent cure for intestinal colic. Barring major injuries the opium was probably used as much for colic as for traumatic pain. The large number of doses of several of the medications was appropriate for a group much larger than the ten to twelve men that Jefferson had suggested. Perhaps Lewis had other ideas and took the precaution of buying enough medicines for a larger group.

Lewis obviously expected to treat venereal disease, and his medical supplies included standard cures such as calomel, copaiba, and mercury. Army officers were responsible for the health of their men, and Lewis and Clark would have been thoroughly familiar with the treatment of venereal disease among soldiers. Mercury, either as a pill or a salve, was the mainstay of most treatment, and it was given until there were signs of mercury intoxication. In addition, syringes for irrigating the penis were included with the other instruments, although no specific mention was made in the journals that they were used.

Lewis could expect to treat all types of wounds and lacerations. It was more than likely that the expedition would get in a fight with the Indians, although the Corps was instructed to avoid confrontations whenever possible. Gunshot and arrow wounds, lacerations from tomahawks and knives, quite apart from the inevitable cuts and bruises they would experience day by day, were the medical problems with which an Army officer would be most familiar. Yellow basilicum, Peruvian bark, and benzoin could all be used to treat superficial wounds and cuts. The small pocket kit of instruments would have contained instruments for probing wounds and removing superficial bullets and arrowheads, but not for stitching lacerations closed. And it was just as well, because closing dirty lacerations without first cleaning them and removing all dirt is a certain road to infection. Leaving a wound open to drain, perhaps packed with a poultice, was standard treatment. In the light of modern knowledge, this treatment was the best under the circumstances. The 2 ounces of lint that Lewis took seem to be very inadequate if it was to be used as a wound dressing or packing, but perhaps they intended to use soft, fluffy, natural substitutes such as cottonwood seeds.

Nutmeg, used now as a pleasant spice for desserts and mulled wine, was regarded as a cure for everything from plague to the "bloody flux," the term then used for bloody diarrhea. Thousands of men died from scurvy, and dozens of ships sank in the search for nutmeg in the Spice Islands. When the Dutch sold Long Island to the British, part of the deal was that the British, in exchange, would give them the Island of Run in the Moluccas where the finest nutmeg trees grew. The reason for nutmeg in the medical kit is not clear, perhaps it was to be used just as flavoring, but 2 ounces would not have lasted long in a group with more than thirty hungry men.

Looking over the list of supplies and equipment Lewis ordered one must be impressed and amazed by the details he thought of, details to ensure success. Guns and rifles were an essential part of the equipment, but guns were no good without powder and balls. Lewis had an ingenious answer to the problem of keeping the powder dry and having enough lead for the balls. He ordered fifty-two lead canisters in which the powder was sealed and kept dry. When a canister became empty it was converted into ammunition. As the expedition progressed the powder remained dry through storms and dunks in the river, and stayed dry in caches and in the miserable cold, wet environment of the West Coast. The Corps never ran out of ammunition and even had enough to give as gifts to the Indians who wanted guns, ammunition, and whiskey more than trinkets and blue beads.

Gifts for the Indians were a major expense, and Lewis did not buy enough. Toward the end, the expedition was down to its last gifts; men sold their own clothes, and Clark bargained medical services to get food and horses. The 30 pounds of beads that Lewis originally packed did not go far. The list of gifts conjures up a picture of Lewis picking through a box of trinkets, wondering what would be suitable for a Chief. The expedition brought 30 calico shirts, East Indian muslin handkerchiefs, red silk handkerchiefs, 144 small cheap mirrors, 288 steels for striking fire, 144 small and cheap scissors, 288 brass thimbles, 288 small knives with brass inlaid handles, 36 pipe tomahawks, 50 pounds spun tobacco, 40 fish gigs, 3 gross fishing hooks, 15 sheets of copper cut into strips 1 inch wide and 1 foot long, 18 brass combs, 24 blankets, 4 dozen finger rings, 12 small medals, and 1 piece red cloth, second quality. There were also medals of various sizes, imprinted with the clasped hands of friendship on one side and President Jefferson on the other. Big medals for important Chiefs; smaller medals for lesser men.

The most expensive item that Lewis purchased was a chronometer for $250 ($5,000 in year-2001 dollars). Jefferson was adamant that one of the results of the expedition would be accurate and precise latitude and longitude measurements at salient spots along the way. The maps that would be made would have to be accurate and a chronometer was essential.

For centuries the computation of longitude had been difficult and inaccurate. Calculations depending on sightings of the planets and stars and the moon could be used, provided the observer had with him the necessary tables. In the 1750s the British government offered a prize equal to about $1 million today to the first person who could find an accurate and reliable way to measure longitude in ships at sea.

There were two methods. One was to calculate longitude from astronomical observations. The other was to calculate the difference in time between the place where the measurement was made and some fixed point. The second method depended on knowing how the measured time differed from the simultaneous time in Greenwich, England. Knowing the number of hours, minutes, and seconds difference between Greenwich and the place where the observation was being made would tell the longitude of that place, because every hour of difference meant 15 degrees of longitude. An expensive chronometer was, therefore, essential. It was a fragile instrument that reacted temperamentally to sand, wind, and rain and needed to be wound every day, a task that Lewis sometimes forgot. As a result, some of the observations were based on fudging the time. Eventually the chronometer gave up the ghost.

Once the buying spree was finished, everything that had been bought was packed in boxes and transported to Pittsburgh where the riverboats were to be built and where the expedition was to start. Lewis left Philadelphia around June 7, 1803, and went to Washington to consult with Jefferson and to get his final orders. The orders were not for Lewis alone, they were also for the Cabinet and members of Congress so that everyone would know how the money they had appropriated would be spent. There was still considerable political opposition to the expedition. Jefferson had to sell the idea, telling some that the expedition would convert the Indians to Christianity, but telling others that the intention was "literary," the code word for scientific. The final instructions, however, made the purposes perfectly clear.

Jefferson completed his revised handwritten instructions for Lewis and Clark by June 20, 1803, two months before Lewis was to leave Washington. Jefferson wanted to know everything that could be observed, measured, and recorded about the country between the Missouri and the West Coast. His instructions were long, clear, and meticulous down to the last detail. The President liked details.

"To Merriwether Lewis, Esquire, Captain of the First Regiment of Infantry of the United States of America. Your situation as the Secretary of the President of the United States has made you acquainted with the objects of my confidential message of January 18th, 1803, to the legislature; you have seen the act they passed which, though expressed in general terms, was meant to sanction those objects, and you are appointed to carry them into execution. . . . The mission of the expedition," he continued later in the long, explicit document, "is to explore the Missouri River, & such principal streams of it, as, by its course and communication with the waters of the Pacific ocean, whether the Columbia, Oregan, Colorado or any other river, may offer the most direct and practicable water communication across the continent for the purpose of commerce." Detailed observations were to be made of the longitude and latitude at many permanent points along the rivers. All the information was to be recorded in journals of which several copies were to be made for security purposes and sent back to Washington.

After asking whether the instruments and equipment necessary had been acquired Jefferson emphasized that the orders also applied if and when the expedition journeyed beyond U.S. territories. At the moment of writing these instructions, the Louisiana Purchase had not been finalized, and it was thought that Lewis would be going through French territory. Secrecy was still important. Jefferson went on to reiterate all the questions Rush had posed and added that, "in all your intercourse with the natives, treat them in the most friendly and conciliatory manner which their own conduct will admit; allay all jealousies as to the cause of your journey, satisfy them of its innocence."

An interesting instruction was to carry "some matter of the Kinepox; inform those of them with whom you may be, of its efficacy as a preservative from the smallpox: and instruct and encourage them in the use of it." Kinepox was cowpox, a disease similar to smallpox, but much milder and not lethal. Scratching a small amount of secretion from a cowpox sore into the skin afforded protection against smallpox. (The word *vaccination* comes from the Latin word for cow, *vacca*.) Jefferson had a strong personal interest in the prevention of smallpox, and he and his family had been vaccinated. Although this suggestion appeared in Jefferson's instructions, the idea had actually been put forward by Attorney General Levi Lincoln, in a letter he wrote to Jefferson on April 14, 1803. "As Capt. Lewis may have in his company, some who have not had the smallpox, would it not be best to carry some of the matter of the kinepox with him?" Lincoln's idea was similar but the purpose was different. He wanted to protect the men of the Corps. Jefferson thought about the political, as well as the medical, advantage of protecting the Indians, hundreds of whom had died from the disease.

Jefferson was also brutally clear about what would happen if the expedition turned into a disaster and all the men were killed. The information so laboriously gained would be lost. "In the loss of yourselves we should lose the information you have acquired. By returning safely with that, you may enable us to renew the essay with better calculated means." In other words, don't get into unnecessary trouble, and if you meet opposition you cannot deal with—back off. Lewis was known as someone who might blunder into a situation rather than back down, so this instruction was a precaution that, as time would tell, would be carefully and skillfully followed.

Jefferson ordered that once the expedition reached the Pacific, contact should be made with a ship that could bring two men back around Cape Horn, carrying with them copies of the journals and specimens. Finally, Jefferson directed that if Lewis was dying or going to be killed, which was a realistic possibility considering the unpredictable behavior of the Indians and the many natural hazards they would meet, he was given authority to appoint a substitute commander in his place.

Lewis was left with no doubt about the purpose of the expedition. It was a military exercise to find a route to the Pacific Ocean, and he was held by oath to follow Jefferson's orders. Lewis was not to make war. He was not to claim land in the name of the United States. He was not to waste time trapping for beaver, searching for valuable minerals, or building permanent forts. He was to find a route to the Pacific Ocean and determine as much about the country along that route as was possible. And, finally, all the observations were "to be taken with great pains and accuracy." Other objectives, such as building trading posts and populating the territory opened by the discoveries, would follow. Likewise, the members of the expedition, with the exception of some river men and hunters who were French Canadians, were all soldiers, receiving military pay. They served under the laws of engagement of the Army and thus were also bound to Jefferson's orders and subject to all the usual punishments for disobedience or mutiny.

Although the journals do not express the feelings explicitly, the shadow of Jefferson continually floated in the background. As Lewis and Clark dealt with the Indians, explored new territory, and planned their future steps, they always knew that their major objective was to return home and report their findings to the President. Onward ho!

THREE

Medicine in 1800

Sir William Osler, a famous Canadian physician, once said in an address to medical students, "Half of what you know today will be discarded fifty years from now. The trouble is, we don't know which half." Meriwether Lewis could not foresee that he was living during an intellectual watershed in medicine, and that within a generation, most of what he had learned from Benjamin Rush would be discarded as nonsense. The Age of Science was just around the corner, but the new road ahead was hard to see. The proponents of the old ways were authoritative and highly respected and did not brook dissension with their ideas.

In the eighteenth and nineteenth centuries doctors were not being trained to think as scientists. They were trained to follow theories that had no experimental backing. There were five medical schools in America, but only a small percentage of men who set up offices as doctors were graduates. Most aspiring doctors became apprentices to well-known practitioners without seeking formal schooling. Some, with less conscience, just advertised themselves as doctors without having had either training or experience. Doctors were not licensed, and anyone could practice medicine; no qualifications were necessary. So, it is not surprising that standards of care varied greatly. Educated physicians such as Benjamin Rush practiced in the big cities. In the countryside family members dispensed most of the medical care, relying on old wives' tales and books about herbal remedies.

Hospitals were miserable, filthy dumping grounds for the disposal of the unwanted—the poor and debtors, those with uncontrollable mental problems, epidemic fevers, and terminal tuberculosis. Nowadays we associate hospitals with surgery and curative treatments. Then, there was no such connection. Surgery was looked down upon as a profession, inferior to the rest of medicine, and was restricted either to simple superficial operations or drastic emergencies such as amputations. Operations were thought of as acts of desperation, associated with war and wounds, not with curing diseases. Surgeons mostly set broken bones and wielded the lancet for opening abscesses or bleeding. Any operation that invaded the body carried with it a horrendous mortality rate from infection. There were, however, occasional glimpses of surgery as we now know it. In 1809 Ephraim MacDowell, a country doctor in Kentucky, successfully removed a 20 pound ovarian tumor from the abdomen of Jane Todd Crawford. McDowell performed the operation on the kitchen table in the patient's home without the benefit of either antisepsis or anesthesia. The patient lived another thirty-one years.

Treatment in 1800 consisted of a large variety of herbs and drugs. Some of these "simples," as the remedies were called, had definite medicinal properties. Others were handed down from generation to generation without providing much benefit, although they did no harm. In addition to minor illnesses and injuries, infections were the major, nonsurgical medical crisis. Learned physicians of the day developed many theories about infections, most without a factual basis. However, some doctors were able to identify specific fevers. A famous seventeenth-century English physician, Thomas Sydenham, recognized that Peruvian bark, the source of quinine, cured only one fever, malaria (known as the "ague"), and had no effect on other infections. Therefore, he concluded that the "ague" was a unique disease unrelated to other fevers. Another physician clearly described the signs and symptoms of typhoid fever and identified it too as a unique disease; once again, a determination based solely on his observations. While some fevers were given names—ague, remittent bilious fever, and so forth—naming the fever did not imply knowledge of a specific cause. Most doctors lumped all fevers into one or two categories and based their treatment on the category into which the fever fell.

Almost all the fevers were due to infections. But, as there was no knowledge of bacteria and how they cause infections, all diseases in which the patient was unusually warm were called a "fever." Fevers were thus diagnosed and treated in several ways. The proponents for one particular theory held very strong views about labeling a fever as either "inflammatory" or "contagious." Fevers that occurred in well-fed, robust people—often country dwellers or rich people— were called "inflammatory." Fevers that developed in poor, thin, ill-fed people living in the cities were likely to be labeled as "contagious." The cause of the fever, by modern standards, did not enter into the diagnosis, which was based on the patient's appearance, the strength of their pulse, the color and smell of their urine, and other observations.

In light of such diagnoses doctors thought that fevers were due to an imbalance between forces within the body. Treatment for some fevers, therefore, corrected excessive internal forces by bleeding or purging to release harmful entities; other sufferers, in whom the forces were believed to be weak, were given stimulants.

In the late nineteenth century scientists began to look for specific bacteria or viruses as causes of each fever, but Benjamin Rush solved the problem of infections in his own mind. For him, not only was there *only* one kind of fever, there was *only* one kind of disease, based on tension in the vascular system, especially of the brain. "I have formerly said that there was but one fever in the world," he once remarked in a lecture to medical students. "Be not startled, Gentlemen, follow me and I will say there is but one disease in the world. The proximate cause of disease is irregular convulsive action in the vascular system affected." This unbelievable concept simplified treatment. If there was only one disease there need only be one cure, and further research was thus unnecessary. Rush's ideas were far off the mark, and his theories of treatment brought scathing comments from his critics.

Rush also believed in "heroic medicine," with bleeding to the point of fainting, and massive purging with doses described as "enough for a horse." John Herdman, however, an Edinburgh physician, wrote in 1803 about influenza: "If you would consider its symptoms in a just and proper point of view, you would find that this method of cure, this evacuatory and antiphlogistic practice, is supported on no good ground whatever: you would draw the lancet with the utmost hesitation, and having done the deed, you would sheath it in fear and trembling." Despite such criticisms, Rush's advice to Lewis continued to encourage bleeding and purging.

To understand Benjamin Rush and his ideas, it is necessary to know more about his life. He was born in 1745, and his father died when he was five years old. His mother was determined that her son should get a good education so he was first sent to the West Nottingham Academy, then to the New Jersey College, the predecessor of Princeton University. At first he intended to enter the law but was dissuaded from this path by Reverend Samuel Davis, the President of the college. Rush was apprenticed to Dr. John Redman, a well-known physician, and worked for five years under his tutelage.

It was common in those days for young physicians who aspired to reach the higher ranks of their profession to study abroad, and Rush was no exception. He went to the University of Edinburgh, one of the most popular European centers for studying medicine. The medical school at Edinburgh had already been teaching students for nearly one hundred years, and its famous teachers attracted many students from America. Men who had studied in Edinburgh started the first medical schools in America, and, of the three physicians who attended George Washington on his deathbed, two were Edinburgh graduates. Rush studied in Edinburgh for two years, and during that time he not only received a medical education that would influence him for the rest of his life, but he made political and social contacts that were almost equally important.

William Cullen, Professor of Medicine in Edinburgh, was the most famous medical teacher of his day and Rush soon attached himself to the doctor's following. Cullen believed that all life is an expression of forces within the nervous system, and that disease is a failure of regulation of those forces. According to Cullen, diminution of the energy of the brain resulted in a "cold fit" and the hot, vasodilated reaction to a fever was a "hot fit." The basis of treatment either was to increase nervous energy with drugs or diet, or reduce it with bleeding, purging, emetics, and semistarvation. Bleeding, purging, and puking were the presumed roads to health, and Rush adopted these treatments in his own practice.

After studying for two years in Edinburgh, Rush graduated M.D. in June 1768. Shortly thereafter, he was granted the Freedom of the City of Edinburgh, an honor that nowadays is only granted to the old and famous, the rich and royalty.

Upon leaving Edinburgh, Rush went first to London, the city of Hogarth and Samuel Johnson, a filthy, exciting, gin-swigging place with huge differences between the lives of the rich and poor. In London, Rush studied under William Hunter, brother of John Hunter, the father of experimental surgical research. There must have been great philosophical differences between Rush and the Hunter brothers. John Hunter once said, "Why think? Why not try the experiment?" Whereas Rush thought that "observation without principles is nothing but empiricism."

Rush returned from Europe in 1769. His practice grew slowly through hard work and attention to his patients, and he taught chemistry at the College of Philadelphia, the first medical school in America.

Rush joined the Army during the Revolutionary War, an experience that also greatly influenced his medical philosophy. After the Battle of Trenton he wrote, "It was now for the first time war appeared to me in its awful plenitude of horrors. I want words to describe the anguish of my soul, excited by the cries and groans and convulsions of the men who lay by my side." Bilious, putrid fevers and smallpox stalked the buildings (they could not be called hospitals) in which as many as one thousand wounded might be crowded. Such experiences could not fail to affect Rush's professional life, his attitude toward his patients, and his concepts of disease.

By the nineteenth century North America was plagued with a devil's cauldron of diseases—measles, diphtheria, trachoma, whooping cough, chicken pox, bubonic plague, malaria, smallpox, yellow fever, cholera, amoebic dysentery, dengue fever, typhus, leprosy, hookworm, mumps, and venereal disease—introduced by Europeans into a continent that had been isolated for millennia. The Indians were not free from diseases and parasitic infestations, but many of the introduced diseases turned out to be disastrous to people whose immune systems were not prepared for the new bacteria. Smallpox, malaria, and venereal diseases exacted a terrible toll of lives and seriously depleted the strength of the native nations. Smallpox, the worst of the plagues, could not be cured and left in its wake only empty, deserted villages and wind-blown graves. Rush's advice to Lewis acknowledged these epidemics in light of the land and peoples that the expedition would visit. Before Lewis and Clark ventured west several devastating epidemics of smallpox had decimated the Indian tribes along the route they would travel. Smallpox was a serious threat to the expedition.

It would be hard to conceive of a worse way to die than from smallpox, then feared more than all the other pestilences sweeping the world. First the patient developed a mild fever, then pain in the chest and a cough, followed by vomiting and a rash. The rash became pustular with oozing sores spreading over the face and the body. High fever wracked the body, and the rash was unendurably irritating making the patient tear at his or her skin and spread infection around the body. As the patient coughed the virus was spread in droplets in the air, so that the unsuspecting attending family became infected. Soon the whole household was infected. Forty percent of smallpox victims died, and those who survived the disease had to live with a disfigured, scarred face. The disease, which has now been eliminated from the world, used to affect and kill millions of people. At the end of the eighteenth century one-third of the population of London was said to carry the scars of the disease. Smallpox virtually eliminated several tribes of American Indians in the early 1800s, and more would share the same fate later in the century. Europe's gift to America was a disaster.

Although smallpox ravaged North America, the Chinese, as early as A.D. 1000, had found a method for preventing the disease. They discovered that if the finely ground substance of a dried scab was puffed up the nose of the person seeking immunity, a mild case of smallpox ensued, followed by lifetime immunity. The same principle of exposing a person to a minor form of the disease was used in variolation, an inoculation procedure termed after the Latin name for smallpox, *variola*. A small amount of the secretion from an active smallpox sore was scraped into the skin of the recipient, and, if all went well, the person only had an attenuated case of smallpox and then acquired immunity. The method was not without danger, and some reports at the time suggested that 12 percent of those treated in this way died, but the treatment became popular in England, Holland, and Germany during the 1700s. The first large-scale attempt to prevent smallpox in the United States took place during the winter of 1777 when General George Washington's troops were encamped at Valley Forge. If smallpox had swept through the Army, the war would have been finished, so Washington had four thousand men inoculated with primitive vaccine taken from mild cases of smallpox. Amazingly, only ten men caught full-blown smallpox and died. Vaccination with cowpox had yet to be discovered.

One discovery, perhaps more than any other, marked the change in Rush's lifetime from old to modern, experiment-based methods of medicine. Edward Jenner was a close friend and former assistant to John Hunter, the founder of scientific experimental surgery. From Hunter, Jenner learned how to develop a hypothesis, design an experiment, and seek the truth through doing rather than thinking.

Jenner was familiar with the myths and stories that circulated among the country people. One story claimed that milkmaids who developed cowpox never became infected with smallpox. Jenner soon found this to be true. He then conceived the following experiment. He would inoculate someone with cowpox and then, later, expose the person to smallpox. On May 14, 1796, he inoculated a small boy, James Phipps, son of a poor farmer, with cowpox and then, six weeks later tried, unsuccessfully, to infect him with smallpox.

Blossom, a cow living deep in the English countryside, was the source of cowpox from which Jenner made the first successful smallpox vaccine. The cow infected her milkmaid, Sarah Nelmes, and Jenner took material from the sores on Sarah's hand and rubbed it into two small cuts on James' arm. A few days later James had the obvious evidence of cowpox: small sores on his skin with a low fever. Six weeks later Jenner variolated James, who should have otherwise developed smallpox. There was no reaction. Nowadays such an experiment would be immoral, unethical, and illegal, but it transformed medicine. Not only had it opened the way to prevent many diseases, but it was a startling example of empirical observation and logical experimentation leading to a definitive result. Two years later Jenner self-published a pamphlet describing his method. President Jefferson received a copy in 1800, three years before the Corps of Discovery began its journey.

Within four years after Jenner published his pamphlet, tens of thousands of people around the world were inoculated with cowpox because several methods were devised to send vaccine from one place to another. A thread could be soaked in the serum from an active cowpock and allowed to dry. The thread was then drawn through the skin of the person to be inoculated. Sharp lancets were dipped in the serum and encased in wax to prevent the vaccine from drying. Active vaccine could also be placed inside small glass capillary tubes and the ends sealed with wax to keep the vaccine fluid. The most successful method in a small community was person-to-person transfer of immunity. One person would be inoculated and, when the pustule became mature in a few days, some of the material was taken and scraped into the skin of the next person, and so on, down the line. Jenner sent the first sample of vaccine for North America (probably in a glass tube or dried on a thread) to a friend, Dr. John Clinch, in Newfoundland in 1800. Later in the same year Dr. Benjamin Waterhouse performed the first smallpox vaccination in the United States and gave vaccine to Thomas Jefferson, who immediately had himself and his whole family protected. It was about this time that Lewis was vaccinated, perhaps with vaccine from the sample sent to Jefferson.

When word got out around the world that there was a wonderful new method of protecting people against the most feared of diseases, doctors everywhere started to demand vaccine. In Europe Dr. Jean de Carro introduced vaccination in Vienna as early as 1799. By 1800, vaccination had spread to Paris and throughout the British fleet in the Mediterranean. A year later it was being administered in Russia under the direction of the widow of Czar Paul I.

There is no indication that Jefferson knew what was happening elsewhere in the world when he urged Lewis to take with him some of the "kinepox." With a wider vision of the possibilities, he would most surely have insisted, rather than suggested, that vaccination be part of the mission. When the British introduced vaccination into

---

While the Lewis and Clark expedition was crossing the continent, a Spanish physician, Francisco Xavier de Balmis, was conducting one of the most remarkable, single-minded crusades in the history of medicine. He had worked for many years in New Spain and had seen many cases of smallpox. After he returned to Spain he persuaded King Charles IV, whose daughter had died from the disease, to allow him to lead an expedition back to the colonies to introduce vaccination. Balmis left Spain in 1803 on a ship carrying twenty-two young orphans as the carriers of vaccine, and the rector of the orphanage. During the voyage the vaccine was passed from child to child. Thirty-nine months later Balmis returned home, having circumnavigated the world. He introduced vaccination to the Canary Islands, Venezuela, Guatemala, Bogota—where more than fifty thousand people were vaccinated—Havana, and across the Pacific to Manila, Batavia, and eventually to Macao in China. Japan excluded all foreigners and vaccination was not accepted there for another fifty years.

India a high authority wrote back to England that this measure had greatly enhanced the popularity of the British government. The same surge of popularity perhaps would have occurred among the American Indians had Jefferson's plan to vaccinate the native population come to fruition. As things turned out, American Indians were frequently afraid of the white man's medicine and often refused vaccination. The one tribe that did accept vaccination, the Sioux, added greatly to their strength by being protected from smallpox.

Fortunately, the Lewis and Clark expedition did not encounter any of the smallpox epidemics that periodically swept through the Indian populations along the Missouri and up the West Coast. If they had found themselves in the middle of an epidemic many of the men would have become infected and the expedition would have imploded, because the men had not been protected. It is surprising that the crew was not protected, because Lewis had been vaccinated and Jefferson was a strong promoter of vaccination, and the efficacy of vaccination was already well accepted.

In addition to smallpox, yellow fever was another plague that caused public panic. When "yellow jack" struck, a long shadow lay across the land. However, this was not a disease that Lewis and Clark were likely to meet. It was restricted to the East Coast ports and the Caribbean. It did, however, play an important part in the history of the Lewis and Clark expedition. It confirmed Rush's view that bleeding and purging were good treatments, and it defeated Napoleon, indirectly bringing about the Louisiana Purchase.

The yellow fever epidemic of 1793 in Philadelphia started on August 5 at the same time that Rush was asked to see the daughter of Dr. Hugh Hodge. She died two days later. Rush's next patient was an old flame, Polly Fisher. He bled and purged her to relieve the symptoms of "bilious remittent fever." She recovered. But by August 24, 150 patients had died.

Rush took to the books to find an appropriate treatment. Sydenham had advised bleeding and purging, so Rush gave his patients several "Thunderbolts" a day. Of the first five patients treated in this way, four survived. Bleeding, according to claims, stopped hemorrhages and vomiting, brought patients out of delirium or coma, and caused the redness of the eyes to disappear. Rush withdrew 114 ounces of blood (7 pints) from one fever patient in five days.

Rush became sick himself and undertook his own cure, bleeding and purging, but he became so weak he could hardly climb the stairs to his patients. "A slow cough fever attended with regular chills and a troublesome cough hung constantly upon me," he recalled, "The contagion now began to affect me in small and infected rooms in the most sensible manner." Four of his pupils and his sister died. Rush took months to recover his own health, but had nonetheless become convinced that bleeding and purging were the cures for yellow fever.

To stop an infectious disease it is more important to know how it is being spread than what is being spread. In 1800 it was clear that some diseases such as smallpox were spread by close contact between infected victims. But the understanding that diseases could be spread from one human to another by an insect vector, such as a mosquito, or through airborne germs was beyond the limits of nineteenth-century knowledge. Contagion and miasmata were the two commonly accepted sources of infection. The notion of contagion was easy to grasp as a cause of disease. People lived close together, and with many cases in the same house, doctors reasoned that diseases were spread from person to person. Miasmata were the mysterious emanations and effluvia from swamps, rotting vegetation, and bad-smelling areas. These fumes and smells seemed to be reasonable sources of disease, especially in a society in which bad smells and open sewers were an accepted part of life. Experimentation, laboratory tests, and microscopic examination were more than fifty years away. Even at the end of the eighteenth century it was unusual to take the temperature of a patient. The clinical thermometer was invented in the seventeenth century but was not used regularly until a Scottish physician, James Currie, began to measure the temperature of his patients. Lewis took three thermometers with him (the last one was accidentally broken in

September 1805), but they were only used for measuring the temperature of the air and water. Although the microscope had been invented, only a dilettante would have owned one and would have used it for amusement rather than the investigation of disease.

The Lewis and Clark expedition could have been exposed to many infectious diseases. Malaria was prevalent in the eastern states and the valleys of the Ohio and Mississippi rivers during the summer months. But it was so common that the public did not fear it in the same way that they feared the unpredictability of smallpox or yellow fever. No one understood the cause of the "ague." It was just accepted as a condition caused by miasmata. By the end of the eighteenth century, malaria was well established along the Mississippi valley. At the time of the expedition, however, it may not have yet reached the Missouri valley.

There were similarities between yellow fever and malaria. Both were imported by the slave trade. Once established, both diseases affected the white population more than the slaves. Plantation owners often explained this by saying that the slaves, being inferior people, were born with intrinsic animal strengths that protected them from diseases. The whites could not realize that slaves coming from West Africa were immune to malaria. It almost became evidence of superior breeding to catch malaria.

The spread of malaria requires two conditions. First, anopheles mosquitoes are necessary to act as transmitters of the parasite. Second, an available reservoir of parasites in the blood of infected humans must be present. Carriers of the malaria parasite, without symptoms, are common in countries where malaria is indigenous. It is, therefore, reasonable to believe that some of the men in the Corps were carriers of malaria. It is conceivable that one of the carriers could have been bitten by an anopheles mosquito, but by the time the parasite had matured in the biting mosquito, the expedition would have been long since gone. The infected mosquito would have flown around and died before being able to infect another person. Spread of the disease to another member of the Corps was extremely unlikely.

Other scenarios were possible. There could already have been parasite-carrying mosquitoes along the river, feeding on infected Indians. But, as the chances of spreading depend on the density both of infected people and infected mosquitoes, given the sparse populations along the Missouri the chances of acquiring malaria would have been very slight.

Could the Corps have spread malaria up the Missouri valley? It is possible, but not very likely. During the earlier part of the journey up the river it might have been theoretically possible for a mosquito to bite an infected member of the Corps and then, a week later, bite an Indian who had never previously been infected. A long shot, but possible. When the Corps was in its winter Mandan camp and stationary for several months, with the best opportunity for the spread of all diseases, there were no mosquitoes to become infected. The same situation applied during the winter of 1805–1806 in Fort Clatsop on the West Coast. Thirty years after the visit of the Corps to the West Coast, malaria played a potent part in the deaths of hundreds of Indians. This outbreak was almost certainly introduced by traders, some of whom had come from China and other malarial areas.

Although they avoided the lethal fevers, many men of the Corps caught venereal diseases. Syphilis and gonorrhea had been accepted as a normal accompaniment of army service for centuries. Lewis made preparations to treat his men because the management of venereal disease was one of the duties of an officer. There were no indications in the journals of unusual annoyance or surprise that some of the men had become infected.

There is still discussion about whether syphilis was introduced into America from Europe or was indigenous to the continent. The sailors of Christopher Columbus brought the disease back with them to Italy, but it is likely that it was already present in Europe, masquerading under a different name. Archaeologists argue about finding the characteristic changes of syphilis in pre-Columbian bones in North America. Lewis suspected that syphilis was an indigenous American disease, but he based his opinion on finding venereal disease in Indians far from white communities. Benjamin Rush, however, was firm in his belief that venereal disease was introduced by Europeans. Regardless, syphilis and gonorrhea were already common and widespread by the time the expedition traveled up the Missouri. Although the area through which the expedition traveled was relatively isolated, there had been many opportunities for infection to be introduced into the Indian population by voyageurs and trappers. The acquiescence of Indian women and the habit of offering women to visiting travelers made spread of the disease inevitable and rapid.

The standard cure of the day was mercury, either taken by mouth or applied locally, as a salve, to the genital lesions. Some of the expedition's men became infected repeatedly, or they had a flare-up of disease they were already carrying. None of the medications they took were curative, but merely suppressed the problems. The Indians had their own herbal cures, of which the root of lobelia (*L. siphilitica*), a purgative and diuretic, was the most widely accepted; but these cures were not used by the men of the Corps. Lewis remarked that many Indians died from, or with, venereal disease, but he did not find that they had any miraculous cures.

Gonorrhea, the "gleet," was common in Europe long before Columbus first visited America. There was no cure, and mercury was more effective against syphilis than against gonorrhea. Gonorrhea in pregnant women can infect the eyes of babies as they pass through the birth canal, and much of the eye disease seen in the Indians by Lewis and Clark was probably gonorrheal.

In addition to venereal diseases, the members of the Corps experienced more than their fair share of diarrhea, but none was due to cholera. Cholera, which was endemic in India for centuries, became a worldwide pandemic in 1817, although it did not invade the United States until 1831.

Much of the white people's medicine was only of limited help to the Indian population, although it was much sought after. It was fortunate for the expedition that they never had to deal with a major epidemic among the Indians with whom they associated, because Lewis and Clark's limited medical skills and resources would have been of little use. None of the Indians who were treated died from the attention they received. But if measles or diphtheria had struck the Indians while the expedition was encamped for either of the winters, the reputation of Lewis and Clark as doctors, even their lives, could have been in jeopardy.

Food also played a major role in health. In the nineteenth century the science of nutrition was unknown. People ate what was available without regard to calories or vitamins. The Corps of Discovery often went through days of privation and became used to a dull, repetitive diet, but no one starved. Scurvy was well recognized by sailors journeying across the oceans and occurred during wars and times of famine. The cause, deficiency of vitamin C, would not be known for a hundred years, but preventing it by consuming vegetables and citrus fruits was already understood. Neither Lewis nor Clark expressed any concern in their journals that the men were showing the signs of scurvy, and as their diet contained fruit and plants, there was no reason they should have become deficient in vitamin C.

Based on the medical concepts of disease in the eighteenth and nineteenth centuries, bleeding, purging, vomiting, and sweating were the mainstays of treatment. Bloodletting now seems to us to be brutal, dangerous, and illogical, but, in 1800, it was regarded as appropriate, beneficial, safe, curative, and the right thing to do. Bleeding had been an accepted treatment for millennia, and was even described by Hippocrates in 400 B.C. And because physicians, including Rush, believed that diseases were caused by evils within the body, many of which resided in the blood, the best way to get rid of those evils was to bleed and purge. The question, obviously, was how much?

To maintain health the volume of blood within the vascular system must be sufficient. The blood must be pumped around the body fast enough to maintain blood pressure and deliver enough oxygen, and there must be enough red cells to carry oxygen. If the first two of these requirements are not met, a person may go into shock. If the third is not met, a person will be anemic.

The bloodletters of old had some serious dilemmas. They could not measure blood pressure, but they could feel the pulse, which is some indication of blood pressure. And they did not know how much blood there was in the body. Their ideas of how much blood was removed may often have been more guesswork than accurate measurement. The "normal" male has about 70 milliliters of blood per kilogram (2.2 pounds) of weight (about 10 pints); the "normal" female, slightly less. Removing about 3 pints from a man results in a sharp drop in blood pressure and fainting. Removal of 4 pints, suddenly, could be fatal if the volume were not replaced quickly.

The standard method for bloodletting was to tie a cloth or tourniquet around the upper arm, sufficiently tight to occlude the veins, but not so tight as to shut off the arterial flow. The veins on the arm swelled up and a sharp lancet was used to nick an engorged vein. Blood flowed into a brass pan used to measure the amount removed. After the desired amount had been removed, the tourniquet was removed and the arm was bandaged to stop the flow. Sometimes this procedure was performed by a doctor, but frequently by an assistant, a phlebotomist, whose job was to bleed patients. On occasion, patients would bleed themselves because there was great public faith in the procedure and because a bloodletter was not always available. Amazingly, patients often exclaimed that they felt better after losing the blood, even after losing a volume great enough to make them faint. Rush frequently advocated bleeding until faintness, and the person was then often bled again the next day. If this was done several times, the patient would be made severely anemic and would take days, if not weeks, to recover a normal red blood cell count.

President George Washington is the most famous patient in American history about whom we know the details of bleeding during his final illness. On December 14, 1799, the President was deathly ill with a severe infection of his throat and pneumonia. He was attended by three physicians, two of whom (James Craik, Gustavus Richard Brown) had trained in Edinburgh and were indoctrinated with a strong belief in the benefits of bleeding. One of them, Dr. James Craik had trained in Edinburgh at the same time as Benjamin Rush. The third physician, Elisha Cullen Dick, younger than the other two, had been trained in Pennsylvania. At 7:30 A.M. Washington was bled 12 to 14 ounces, about 1 pint, and asked that he be bled more. At 9:30 A.M. he was bled another pint and a half, and again at about 11:00 A.M. After a little while, he felt well enough to get out of bed and walk in the bedroom. During the afternoon Dr. Dick, the youngest physician, argued that Washington would be weakened by more bleeding. Nevertheless, another 2 pints were removed at 3:00 P.M. At 4:00 P.M. the President was given a laxative and an emetic. (While this drama was unfolding, Rush, the dominant advocate for bleeding, was awaiting the verdict in a trial in Philadelphia in which he had sued a critic for accusing him of excessive bloodletting.)

Washington improved briefly but was still acutely breathless. His doctors discussed, but decided against, tracheotomy. Washington, sensing that he was near death, examined his will and left instructions for his burial. At 10:20 P.M., he died. He had been bled 80 ounces (2,365 milliliters; 5 pints) in twelve hours. The cause of Washington's death has been argued from the day he died, but that he was bled half his blood volume over twelve hours while he was so seriously ill can have had nothing but a deleterious effect on the outcome.

Bleeding and purging continued to be the mainstays of treatment for most diseases, although by the 1820s and 1830s the tide was turning against such "heroic" measures. In the 1850s Louis Pasteur's discovery of germs and the advent of scientific methods of looking at disease brought this era to an end, although there were still advocates for bleeding at the time of the Civil War. Bleeding is still used for a very few specific diseases such as polycythemia, in which there is an excess of red cells in the blood, rendering the blood viscous and slow to circulate. Now medical practice has moved full circle, with blood being stored and separated into its valuable components to replace what has been lost through trauma, surgical operations or disease.

It is not surprising that Benjamin Rush requested Lewis to find out about the diseases afflicting the Indians and the native cures.

Rush believed that the diseases of America differed from those of Europe, and that the only disease afflicting the Indians was fever, a composite disease with many causes. The Indians certainly suffered from many different fevers, but they also suffered from digestive disorders, rheumatism, respiratory problems, arthritis, and scurvy. Tuberculosis was present but was not common. Neurologic and mental diseases, arteriosclerosis, and cancer were rare. The rarity of mental disturbances among the Indians was ascribed to the closeness of family life and the support and comfort available within the structure of their society. Even in the seventeenth century a suggestion was made that the stress of Indian life was less than that for the whites because the Indians had no lawsuits and were burdened by fewer possessions.

The early settlers praised the health and physique of the Indians who were strong of limb, fleet of foot, and seemingly had few diseases. Some of the comments written at the time confirmed that impression. "Very rare to see a sick body among them." "Never did see one that was born in either defect or endurance a monster . . . save one that had a bleared eye." The tall, lean men able to hunt the deer and grow the crops they needed, free from many of the diseases so familiar to the settlers, must have seemed remarkably healthy. Perhaps they were. Over the centuries the Indians had acquired their good health through natural selection. Among the nomadic tribes, strong limbs and the ability to keep up with the group were essential. The weak and unfit died. The Indians lived in harsh environments and were capable of enduring extreme hardship and privation. Famine alternated with feast, drought with flood, forest fire with lush greenness, peace with war. The cycles of life were accepted, if not always with quiet acquiescence, at least with an understanding that every generation faced the same tribulations.

The Indians had discovered their own medicines over thousands of years, choosing natural cures from the profusion of plants that grew around them. The plants they selected varied from area to area and from tribe to tribe, but there was a remarkable similarity between the groups of agents: cathartics, emetics, febrifuges for dispersing fevers, vermifuges for dealing with intestinal worms, drugs for pain, ointments for wounds and burns, and agents to control the pain of childbirth. The troubles and infirmities of humanity remained the same regardless of tribe or race.

Many plants were chosen because they looked like the disease they were supposed to cure. A yellow plant would be chosen to cure jaundice, a red plant to cure a problem with the blood, a twisting plant for snakebites. Ill-tasting, bitter plants were believed to cause evil spirits to leave the body. Others were chosen because, by good luck or serendipity, they were found to cure a specific problem. No one knows, for instance, who first tried the quinine-rich bark of the cinchona tree as a cure for malaria. By the time the first white person was given the bark the natives had used it for centuries. The Indians soon realized that some of the cures offered by white doctors were superior to their own, although the results did not always impress the Indians. The complete failure of the whites to cure smallpox and other plagues must have diminished the reputation of the foreigners' cures.

The Indians believed that diseases were the result of natural, supernatural, or human causes. Natural and human causes were plain. But all was not that simple. An apparently "natural" event could be caused by supernatural intervention or result from an improper ritual in the handling of a killed animal, or the breaking of a taboo. If the right prayer was not said when a deer was killed, the leg broken on the way back to camp might be attributed to the enraged spirit of the deer.

The medicine man or shaman played an important part in the conduct of healing ceremonies. He was more of a priest than a healer. Many of the healers were women who laid on hands, massaged the injured, and concocted the medicinal potions. The shamans were the medium through whom the spirits could be urged to heal. Medicine men could also remove unruly spirits from those with illnesses. Rituals, songs, and dances were an essential part of the cures. Some of what they did was pure fakery, but much—although perhaps they did not realize it—was applied psychotherapy.

Many diseases were thought to be due to intrusion either of objects or animals into the body. This theory laid itself open to fraud because an unprincipled shaman could easily convince someone that a snake had entered his or her body. Then, in the course of a complicated ritual, through sleight of hand, he could produce a small garter snake from the person's body. There is nothing new or original about this trickery. Quacks all over the world still play similar conjuring tricks on unsuspecting victims.

The tools of the trade for the shamans were skins and bones, feathers and animal skins, drums and rattles—quite different from the lancets and laxatives of their white counterparts. Through these tools, power was imparted to the patient and to the medicinal plants the sick person received. There were specific songs, dances, and prayers for every disease. The correct use of these was the responsibility of the shaman. When the word *medicine* was spoken, it really meant *mystery*. Things that were described as "big medicine" were those full of mystery.

Indian medical practice sometimes differed sharply from that of the whites. For instance, the Puritanical, Calvinistic settlers believed that childbirth should be painful, but the Indians believed that the pain of childbirth should be relieved. A tea made from snakeroot or fried onions mixed with olive oil assured a painless birth. Drinking the ground-up rattle of a rattlesnake was also a source of pain relief used by the Choctaws. Sacagawea received a similar mixture during the delivery of her child. Most Indian women delivered their children quickly and with remarkably little interruption of their lives. The babies were "delivered in a trice with not so much as a groan."

Childbirth and menstruation, however, were not without taboos. Menstruating Indian women were segregated in special huts and were not allowed social contacts for several days. In many tribes a girl's first menstrual period was a cause for celebration because it showed she had reached the age for marriage and pregnancy. The Chinooks surrounded pregnancy with many taboos and superstitions. The mother-to-be could not sleep long, she could not lie in the sun, she could not wear jewelry, and she must not look on the dead. Diet was strictly controlled. No trout. No food with a hole in it. To look at a dog whose eyes were closed would mean that the child would be born blind. Even the husband's behavior was similarly constrained. He could not kill raccoons or otters, he could not shoot a bird or cast eyes on a corpse. Breaking one of these taboos could mean the birth of a deformed child or its early death.

Nutritional problems must have been common in Native Americans. The failure of a harvest, a drought, or floods would wreck havoc with people who usually could grow and store just enough food for a single season. Scurvy was well recognized. The Indians knew that as winter progressed and spring approached, people could grow weak, their gums might bleed, and their teeth become weak in the sockets. They also knew that eating certain green plants early in spring would result in a quick cure.

When Jacques Cartier, a French explorer, and his ships were trapped in the ice of the Saint Lawrence River in the winter of 1535 and 1536, his sailors became deathly sick with scurvy. The local Indians also became sick but were cured by drinking tea made from the leaves of a tree. Cartier immediately had the tea made, but his fearful sailors at first refused to drink it, supposing that it might be poisonous. But those who did drink became better after taking the tea only two or three times. Cartier said that "all the doctors of Louvain and Montpellier could not have done as much in a year as this tree did in eight days."

The Indians based most of their treatments on plants. There were no minerals in their pharmacopoeia (with the exception that some tribes in western Pennsylvania mixed petroleum into their ointments) and few animal products were used except fat from various species, usually in ointments. Wildcat, raccoon, buffalo, and even rattlesnake fat all found their way into assorted liniments. Various writers of the time described anywhere from forty-five to two hundred plants used by the Indians for medicinal purposes. Cascara sagrada, podophyllin, and jalap from Mexico became

popular cathartics with the whites and remained in their pharmacopoeia from many years. Lewis included jalap in his medical kit,
and it was also used by Thomas Jefferson to cure the bowel spasms
from which he seemed to suffer.

Plants such as peyote were used to achieve what we would now
call a "high," but most Indians did not ferment plants for alcohol.
After the whites introduced alcohol to the Indians, drunkenness
soon became a problem. There were, however, standout tribes that
did not use alcohol. When Lewis and Clark reached the Arikaras
on the Missouri and offered the traditional drams of whiskey, they
were quickly refused. Why, the Arikaras asked, would anyone
want to drink anything that so quickly addled their brains? The
Clatsops, on the West Coast, also did not drink alcohol. When
Lieutenant William Broughton of the Royal Navy made his first
landing in 1792 along the Columbia, he offered alcohol to the
Chinooks. They became so upset by the sensations of intoxication
that their people never took alcohol again.

Legend has it that the earliest Jesuit missionaries in Peru were
told of a magical drug that could cure the "ague." In 1632 Father
Alonso Messias brought the drug to Rome—a hotbed of malaria—
where it was soon acclaimed for its miraculous properties in curing
a disease that had defied all other medications. Quinine—Peruvian
bark—had been in use as a general febrifuge for two centuries
before the Lewis and Clark expedition. It was recognized as specific for the intermittent fever of malaria, but because malaria was
not clearly distinguished from other febrile afflictions "the bark"
was often given for fevers in which it could not be effective.
Quinine is still used for the treatment of malaria cases resistant to
other, more modern medications.

Sassafras was also given for many complaints: for fevers, venereal
disease, tuberculosis, and kidney stones, and it was placed on
wounds and bruises as a poultice. So popular was this plant that, at
one time, sassafras and tobacco were the two major exports from
Virginia. Sage tea, sarsaparilla, feverfew, ginseng, and chamomile were
some of the many other plants given by the Indians to treat fevers.

Poisonous snakes are widespread throughout the United States, and as most Indians lived where snakes were common, thousands of bites must have occurred every year. Their supposed cures were numerous. Poultices to rub on the bite. Concoctions of plants to swallow. Charms to keep snakes away. Plantains, hog's lard, the body of the snake cut up and applied to the bite. The cures were limited only by the imagination of the user. Benjamin Barton, a distinguished Philadelphia botanist and an advisor to Lewis, investigated more than thirty Indian cures for snakebites and came to the conclusion that not one of them was of any value. He did, however, believe that the Indian method of applying a tourniquet, incising the bite, and sucking out the poison had merit. It is only in the past few years that the efficacy of this method has been questioned.

Cupping and suction were used for general aches and pains as well as for removing obvious poisons. The shaman would suck vigorously on the affected limb, sometimes apparently sucking blood through intact skin. Hollow bones and reeds were used to suck out poisons from wounds. The principle was always the same: pain is due to a cause within the body that can be removed. If it could not be sucked out directly, a small incision over the painful area would make the removal of the cause easier.

Some Indian tribes used phlebotomy, or bleeding, but not with the wild enthusiasm of Benjamin Rush and his white colleagues. The technique may have been learned from white physicians. Sometimes the blood loss was minimal, being produced by scarification over a painful area with a sharp flint or the fangs of a snake. Obsidian flakes, which can be sharpened to an edge only a few atoms across, were tied to wooden handles and used as lancets after a tourniquet of deer hide had been tied loosely around the limb to engorge the veins.

Although the Indians were skillful in dealing with injuries, little is known about their techniques for closing lacerations and wounds. They often irrigated wounds with a syringe made from a hollow quill and a bladder (a thoroughly modern, effective technique and much safer than suturing a dirty wound) and then bound a poultice over the injury. External wounds and lacerations are one thing, but deep wounds involving the body cavities are a totally different surgical challenge. There were reports that some Indians knew how to deal with chest wounds, but it is hard to believe that there were more than occasional lucky successes.

Sweating was one of the most ancient healing techniques used throughout the Americas. John Smith, in the first Virginian colony, described a sweat house built in the shape of a domed English dove house, in which the Indians placed heated stones in a pot. Sweating was used for cleansing, curing, and for religious ceremonies. Sometimes a session in the sweat house was followed by a plunge into cold water, as is nowadays common after time in the sauna, but the cold plunge was believed to be especially harmful to people with tuberculosis.

By the time of the Lewis and Clark expedition the herbalism of white and Indian medicines had become intermingled. The whites, especially those living in remote areas without access to doctors, had no sources of medical knowledge other than their own folk medicine, mixed with what they had learned from the Indians. The Indians, in their turn, had learned from the whites. When Benjamin Rush asked Lewis to inquire about Indian cures he probably had a good idea that nothing dramatically new would be found unless it was from some tribes that had never been in contact with white traders and explorers.

Indian medicine almost certainly had more to contribute than has been passed down through the generations. Modern pharmaceutical firms are now spending millions of dollars searching the jungles and testing plants for new cures. The white invaders and settlers were, on the whole, not very receptive to Indian ideas and treatments, often scoffing at them as primitive and pagan. The native people, however, survived for thousands of years, treating themselves with their own simples. A few observers recognized they had knowledge to contribute that was clearly effective and should be passed on. But we do not know what was lost and will never be recovered.

FOUR

Pittsburgh to the Mandans:
August 1803–November 1804

The start of the Lewis and Clark expedition was not auspicious. Lewis had struggled for several weeks in Pittsburgh to get his keelboat built by a procrastinating, drunken shipwright. Finally, on August 30, 1803, accompanied by eleven men, including a pilot and three men who hoped to be permanent members of the group, Lewis started down the Ohio River.

Three miles downstream, at Bruno's Island, the party pulled ashore to greet friends and well-wishers. Some of the men present wanted to try Lewis' new air gun, which did not require powder to fire. A Mr. Blaze Cenas—an appropriate name—took the gun, with which he was not familiar, and promptly fired it. A shriek rose from a lady about 40 yards away as the ball went through her elaborate hat, worn especially for the occasion, and sliced across her head. She fell to the ground, blood pouring from a superficial scalp wound. Fortunately, the ball had only grazed her skull and "by examination we found the wound by no means mortal or even dangerous." The sentence in Lewis' journal continued with only a comma, "called the hands aboard and proceeded to a ripple of McKee's Rock." So much for the unfortunate lady with a bloody head and a hat with a hole through it. She was mentioned no more. If she had been killed the start would have been further delayed, and who knows what legal entanglements might have ensued. Good luck, which was to play an important part in the success of the expedition, shone on them from the first day.

That night Lewis made a note in his journal that was going to strike a familiar tune during the next three years. "Halted for the night much fatiegued after laboring with my men all day . . . gave my men some whiskey and retired to rest at 8 o'clock."

The next days and weeks were hard work and little fun. The river was extremely low, and the crew was constantly jumping overboard to push and lift the boat over obstructions or hauling it through shallow water and over sandbars. In places, riffles and rapids threatened to overturn the boat. The boat sometimes became so stuck that horses or oxen were hired to pull it into deeper water. Progress was slow, and Lewis must soon have realized that any hope of starting the ascent of the Missouri before winter set in was fading fast.

Not all the settlers along the shore were helpful. Many travelers probably asked for aid, and, as far as those on shore were concerned, this was just another government group that did not know how to get themselves down the river. Lewis thought the charges for help were excessive and the helpers lazy.

There were unending details to be attended to along the way. A canoe that accompanied them leaked, and valuable gifts for the Indians became wet and had to be repacked in oiled-cloth bags. The iron articles—guns, tomahawks, and knives—rusted and had to be cleaned, placed in the sun, and oiled before being repackaged.

During this time Lewis recorded very little illness in the men. Considering the strenuous nature of their work there must have been cuts and bruises, muscle strains, and sore backs. But the men were used to hard work, and minor complaints were not worthy of description in a journal that had weightier matters to record.

On September 8 the Captain called a halt for a day of rest. While ashore and dining with a Colonel Thomas Rodney, Lewis met Dr. William Patterson, son of a Professor of Mathematics at the University of Pennsylvania, with whom he had consulted before starting on the voyage. Dr. Patterson, Jr. was very anxious to join the expedition as a doctor. Lewis had the authority to recruit someone of this position and said Patterson could come, provided he could be ready by 3:00 the next afternoon. Whether this tight schedule was a way to discourage Dr. Patterson is not clear, but 3:00 P.M. came and went and there was no Dr. Patterson. And it was just as well, for Patterson was a chronic alcoholic and probably would have been a nuisance at least, and a useless encumbrance at worst.

One companion that Lewis valued over almost all others was his dog, a Newfoundland. The name of the dog has been variously translated as Scammon or Seaman, and it seems as though the latter name is correct, the first name being a misinterpretation of poor handwriting. The Indians, used to the scrawny animals that hung around their camps, were very impressed by this large and friendly black dog that obeyed commands and swam better than a person. One Indian offered three beaver skins for the dog, but Lewis, who valued the dog for its good temperament and watchdog skills, wrote, "and of course there was no bargain, I had given $20 for this dog." As any dog lover knows, ten times that amount would not have bought the companion that eventually survived the whole trip.

In the middle of November Lewis had an attack of fever, which he described as the "ague," the shivering that precedes the fever of malaria. He did not take a dose of Peruvian bark, which would

---

Lewis was obviously very fond of his dog that became an important guardian, chasing away wolves, bears, and buffalo. He was a good hunter, diving under the water to catch beaver. On one occasion he was severely bitten by a beaver, and Lewis was afraid the dog would bleed to death. Interestingly enough, one of the few occasions on which Lewis ordered his men to fire on Indians was when Seaman was stolen and a party was sent to retrieve him. They were ordered to shoot, if necessary, to recover him. Lewis stopped writing his journal before the end of the expedition and Seaman's fate is a matter for conjecture.

have been logical, but purged himself with a dose of Rush's Thunderbolts, which operated extremely well and the fever stopped. Lewis must have been familiar with the symptoms of malaria and had probably suffered from it on several occasions. If so, it is strange that he relied more on purging than the bark that was known to be a cure for the "ague."

Lewis met up with Clark at Clarksville in the Indiana Territory later in November. Clark had already recruited nine young men from Kentucky, all experienced backwoodsmen and hunters, who joined the boat as it headed up the Mississippi toward St. Louis. At Cape Girardeau Lewis went ashore, as he frequently did, leaving others to manage the boat. He found the local Commandant to be away at the horse races, where he was responsible for settling arguments between the winners and losers, as well as taking part in the races. On returning to the boat Lewis found Captain Clark "very unwell." This brief entry in the journal is typical of many, both intriguing and exasperating to the inquirer interested in the illnesses of the group. No further mention was made of Clark's progress in subsequent days, and the nature of the illness remains a mystery.

On November 28, Lewis took a reprieve from making any entries in the journal and left Clark in charge of the boat to continue on up the river. During the subsequent years Clark was a much more faithful keeper of the journal than Lewis. Sometimes Lewis was away on a separate venture, but often he just failed to write. The reasons for these long gaps are not clear. Some historians have ascribed the pauses to psychological reasons, and one author has said that during these periods Lewis was in a "blue funk," an unkind portrayal of a singularly courageous man. Depressed, indisposed, distracted, or absent he may have been—but he was never in a blue funk.

Clark's entries tended to be shorter, more precise, and less lyrically descriptive than Lewis'. He was extraordinarily faithful in making the entries, and we would be in a sorry situation in knowing about the details of the journey had he not kept such a detailed, day-by-day diary. In many instances the entries by Clark and Lewis are almost identical. Jefferson had urged that they keep copies so that if one was destroyed, the other would survive. In addition, others were urged to keep journals, and four of the crew—Sergeants Charles Floyd, John Ordway, and Joseph Whitehouse, and Corporal Patrick Gass—recorded journals that provide additional details and viewpoints.

By December 12, 1803, the Corps had reached the Wood River, a tributary of the Mississippi north of St. Louis and opposite the mouth of the Missouri. Here they set up camp for the winter. They chose a place to build huts, and Clark set the men to clearing the land and cutting down trees for the buildings. They had come prepared for this. Not only did they have the equipment for felling and trimming trees, but they had skilled carpenters. Almost all the men, being backwoodsmen, knew how to build a cabin, how to cut the trees and lay out the plan, how to put in the windows and doors, and how to chink the gaps between the logs with moss and mud to make a tight, wind-and-rainproof home.

Almost immediately the journal entries reflected the life they were leading. Indians came to visit bringing meat to sell. The Corps' own hunters shot grouse, turkeys, and deer. Clark started to record the daily temperature and weather conditions, and the precise longitude and latitude of the camp was recorded.

On their first Christmas, Clark was awakened by a discharge of arms. Some of the party were already drunk and "the men frolicked and hunted all day." Perhaps the most important event that day was that George Drouillard—usually called Drewyer in the journals— finally agreed to the terms of his employment (he was not an Army man). He turned out to be the most valuable person in the group after Lewis and Clark themselves. A superb hunter and woodsman, he was able to supply meat for the Corps when others brought home nothing, and whenever a dangerous task called for special skill Drouillard was always chosen.

The winter was cold with hail and snow, and ice flowed down the river. The huts were not finished until some weeks had passed, but the men were allowed out of camp to hone their shooting and hunting skills and release their frustrations. Local white settlers and Indians visited and indulged in shooting competitions and gambling and usually lost both the competition and their money. As the months passed and the weather improved, Clark's recordings told of approaching spring, returning geese and swans, the first emerging garter snake, and the first muskrat.

At the Wood River Camp Clark chose and trained the expedition's final crew. Discipline was sometimes a problem. Men sneaked out of camp to find whiskey and were punished when they were caught. When the Captains left the camp Sergeant John Ordway was in charge, but many of the men disobeyed his orders. John Shields opposed Ordway and threatened his life. William Warner and John Potts fought. So did John Newman and John Colter. Most of the offenders regretted their misbehavior and returned to favor. If Clark had sent them packing, he might not have been able to find others to take their places. The whole expedition could have been in jeopardy.

There were few health problems during the winter of 1803–1804 and none was serious. Clark remarked on his own health—"very sick," "very unwell," "take physick," "sick all night." But we never learn the true nature of his sicknesses. He was "sick" for four days in a row and may have had "flu" or an intestinal upset, but as "physick," a general term for a laxative, was a cure for almost every illness, the treatment did not give a clue to the nature of the illness. Clark was sick more often than anyone else, but there were probably many occasions when others did not feel well and failed to mention it. When Sergeant Nathaniel Pryor became sick Clark had squirrel soup made for him to settle his stomach. Another man had rheumatism, but considering that most of the men were hunting and constantly moving through the woods, building huts, and preparing the boat for the voyage, it is surprising that we do not read of lacerations, sprains, and dislocations. Overall, the health of the group was remarkably good.

In April the journal was full of the details of preparation. Clark measured out the keelboat and one of the dugout canoes, called a pirogue—the "white" pirogue that eventually went all the way to the Great Falls—and calculated how the men and baggage would fit in. There were long lists of the crew and the Sergeants (see Appendix A), the divisions into squads and messes, and details of food: 4,175 complete rations @14 cents—$605.37; 5,555 rations of flour @ 4 cents—$231.97; 100 gallons of whiskey @ 128 cents per gallon; and another 20 gallons of whiskey for $25. The total cost for food was $1,376.85 (about $27,345 today). Most of these rations were not expected to last for the whole trip. As a resupply was impossible the leaders must have known that they would have to find substitute items, or go without.

Clark made out different lists on different days as though he was remembering items day by day. Some lists were for large items— kegs of flour and pork. Others were for very small items—1 bag of coffee, 7 bags of biscuits, 1 bag candle wax, 2 boxes candles. At the end of one list was the brief entry, "Several men for Drunkness today, wind very hard."

On April 30 Clark could record, "a fair day. All hands at work. Mr. Hay nearly finished up packing goods." The time for departure was growing close and the sense of excitement must have been rising in the camp, although the journal entries did not reflect the change in atmosphere. Men got drunk. They wrote letters. The food was re-examined, and some of the pork already packed was condemned. Final orders were given to the Sergeants. The locals came into camp to indulge in shooting competitions with the usual result. "All visitors get beet [sic] and lose their money." Still, no major health problems arose.

May 8, 1804: After loading the keelboat and manning it with twenty oarsmen they went into the middle of the river and rowed a few miles up the Mississippi. It was a successful test run. The next day the men were moved into tents, and Clark sent some of them across the river to the Missouri to collect drinking water that was much cooler than that in the Mississippi. The men were ordered to prepare 100 balls each for their rifles and 2 pounds of buckshot for their muskets. Life was becoming serious.

The weather became hotter and rainy. A final message was sent to Lewis, who had stayed behind in St. Louis to finish some business, telling him that all was set. The keelboat and the pirogues were loaded and complete with sails, and all the men had their ammunition. "Boats and everything complete" was the message. The Corps, "composed of robust helthy [sic] hardy young men" was ready to leave.

Embarking by boat has a certain glamour and excitement that cannot be compared with other departures. Clark was a down-to-earth man who wrote the entries in his journal without many frills. Somehow he managed to make their departure sound like a walk around the block to the store, without the usual fanfare that many departures warrant and receive. The first entry for May 14, 1804, was brief. "Monday 14th a cloudy morning fixing for a start Some provisions on examination found to be wet . . . rain at 9 o'clock . . . I set out at 4 o'clock to the head of the first island in the Missourie 6 miles and . . . incamped, on the island . . . rained." The next day Clark made a slightly more descriptive entry: "Set out from Camp River at Dubois at 4 o'clock P.M. and proceeded up the Missouri under sail to the first Island in the Missouri and camped . . . men in high spirits." "Under sail" conjures up a vision of a square rigged ship leaving port, with cheering people lining the decks—quite a cause for celebration.

Captain Lewis was still in St. Louis. So, Clark sailed a few miles farther to St. Charles, a small French settlement with one hundred houses and about 450 people, where the local people ran out onto the banks to greet them. While Clark went ashore to dine with a local worthy, three men of the Corps were confined for misbehavior. A court-martial was immediately convened to try Warner, Hugh Hall and John Collins for being absent without leave, for behaving in an unbecoming manner, and for speaking in derogatory terms about their superiors. One can easily imagine what three drunken soldiers said about their Sergeant when he reprimanded them for staggering in late after a dance. The punishment for Collins was fifty lashes on his naked back, plus, presumably, a monstrous hangover. The punishments for Warner and Hall were remitted on the recommendation of the court, which was composed of their fellow soldiers.

On May 20 Lewis, accompanied by a number of respectable citizens of St. Louis, set out on horseback "in order to join my friend and companion Capt. William Clark who had previously arrived at that place with the party destined for the discovery of the interior of the continent of North America." Talk about confidence!

Lewis arrived at St. Charles in a shower of rain. The rain was still falling at 3:00 the next afternoon, when, to a shout of three cheers from the locals on the bank, the expedition proceeded for another 3 miles and camped. They were still not completely free, for three of the French boatmen had to go back to town to complete some unfinished business of an undisclosed nature. On May 22 the expedition was finally on its way.

In spite of the rain it must have been a gallant scene. The little armada consisted of the keelboat, a substantial vessel, and two pirogues. The keelboat was 55 feet long, with a beam of 8 feet and a mast 32 feet high. There was a 10-foot elevated deck at the stern that contained a cabin, and another 10-foot deck at the bow. Between the decks were eleven benches for the oarsmen, each bench with enough room for two men: the whole arrangement reminiscent of an ancient Roman galley. The pirogues were large canoes with masts to accommodate a sail. They could carry a considerable load and required several men to paddle them. Being of shallow draft and without a keel they were not stable and needed skill and experience to handle them. As the men pulled away from the shore, the oars slapping the water, dipping and rising, the flag flapping at the stern, many a spectator must have turned to a neighbor and wondered if they would ever see the Corps again.

Twenty-two Army Privates were assigned to row the keelboat, with three Sergeants and the two Captains. Six Privates and Corporal Richard Warfington manned one of the pirogues, and the crew of the other pirogue consisted of six French engagés, all experienced river experts. One of the French crew, Pierre Cruzatte, who would later play an important part in a major crisis of the voyage, was a good fiddler, and on many occasions Lewis called upon him to strike up a tune and set the men "a-dancing."

At their first camp the Indians greeted the Corps and promised them food. They received four deer in exchange for two quarts of whiskey. The next day more Indians brought more deer, and received more whiskey. At this rate of exchange even the 120 gallons of whiskey they had brought would not last long.

Setting sail again, they soon encountered the hazards of the river that would be a constant threat for hundreds of miles. The Missouri, or "Big Muddy" as it was called, was a huge, opaque, roiling river, constantly changing its course. The banks were soft and easily eroded by the current, and sailing close to the shore was dangerous because masses of sand and earth could suddenly collapse on a passing boat. Small branches, logs, and whole trees were swept along, bobbing and dipping in the swirling water, sinking beneath the surface then rising suddenly to crash into a boat. Trees on the bank that had been undermined by the current fell into the water with their roots still held firm and swayed back and forth in the current like giant sweeps. The cumbersome, flat-bottomed keelboat was not maneuverable enough to get out of the way of every obstruction, and a Sergeant stationed at the bow had to warn of every danger.

Sometimes the river was deep enough for rowing. In other places the men had to pole the keelboat—standing on the side decks, punting in unison with their poles. As the pole of the man at the stern came off the bottom, he ran to the bow and started pushing again—a constant circuit of men moving from bow to stern. In some places the river was so shallow the men had to jump overboard and push and lift the boat—loaded with several tons of gear—over a sandbar, or haul the boat by a cordelle, a rope attached to the bow and the mast. And, to top it off, not all the men could swim. On several occasions men who fell into the stream were in great danger of drowning. The wind was as fickle and dangerous as the current. A good upstream wind allowed the men to set the sail and progress with speed. But if the boat, in full sail, turned beam on to both wind and current it could easily capsize, a near disaster that happened more than once. Not only could lives have been lost, but valuable equipment and supplies could have sunk to the bottom of the river, jeopardizing success. To avoid this disaster, the important supplies were shared between the keelboat and the two pirogues. The pirogues were more stable and manageable, but like any canoe, could capsize.

Only two days up the Missouri, Clark wrote: "The swiftness of the current wheeled the boat, broke our Toe rope and was nearly over Setting the boat, all hands jumped on the upper side and bore on that side until the Sand washed from under the boat." Anyone familiar with white-water rafting knows well the cry "High side!" when the raft threatens to keel over. Everyone hurls themselves to the high side to prevent an upset—hard enough in a rubber raft, a different matter in a 55-foot wooden boat swinging out of control in a stretch of the river called the Devil's Race Ground.

On another occasion the keelboat struck an underwater snag that turned it into a "disagreeable and dangerous situation." The men leaped overboard to pull the boat off the hazard. The situation was saved and that evening Lewis wrote in his journal, with some pride, "I can say with confidence that our party is not inferior to any that was ever on the waters of the Missoppie [sic]."

One day, while walking on shore, Lewis climbed a small hill and, on the way down, slipped and nearly fell off a cliff, saving himself by digging his knife into the earth. This was not the only time Lewis came close to a serious accident. He often walked or rode along the shore, exploring and recording the sights, the plants, and the animals. He had encounters with dangerous animals and, in some places, could have met hostile Indians. He was often far from the rest of the group. Had he been injured help would have been slow in coming, and he might not have been found. The question of allowing the Captain of the expedition to endanger himself does not seem to have arisen. The side trips that Lewis made were not just for pleasure. The banks of the river were often so high that it was impossible to get a sense of the country from the river. By climbing up the bluffs or going through the woods along the banks Lewis could look out over the prairies, figure out the lay of the land, and scout for Indians or game. The bottomlands were thick with cottonwoods, the first trees to reseed after the floods that constantly changed the course of the river—a river that was described as the hungriest in the land, sometimes eating 80 acres in a single bite from the banks.

The Corps of Discovery saw a land virtually untouched by humans, with limitless space, clean water uncontaminated by industrial waste, air that sparkled with clarity, and animals and fish in numbers beyond counting and imagination. The land was the home to hundreds of species of migrating birds, animals, and reptiles. The rivers were filled with 150 species of fish. One day white feathers adorned the river in a thick carpet for mile after mile. Finally, as the boats rounded a bend the cause became obvious: thousands of white pelicans on the sandbars were preening themselves, their feathers floating away in the wind and landing on the water. "For three miles after I saw those feathers," Lewis wrote, "we did not perceive from whence they came, at length we were surprised by a flock of Pillican at rest on a sand bar." As the summer passed into fall, long skeins of geese, sandhill and whooping cranes, and swans and ducks flew high overhead migrating south and filling the night sky with haunting song.

Despite the beauty, life on the river was tough and often traumatic. The men were constantly in and out of the water. Sometimes the sun shone and burned their backs, or the rain lashed down and soaked them. The ropes rubbed their hands raw, and their clothes soon wore out. Boots were forgotten and replaced by moccasins. On shore there were cactuses, sharp sticks, and stones to cut their feet. Boils—"tumors and imposthumes"—were common. There has been much discussion about the frequency of boils and the reasons for them. Were the men's immune systems somehow compromised by a poor diet? They were constantly in the water. Was there something in the water that infected them? The water was muddy and filthy and, in places, contaminated with carcasses of animals and the effluvia from Indian villages. Lewis mentioned soap only once in his lists of supplies, and washing was probably a low priority. Washing was not regarded as a healthy habit, even in polite city society. So, it would not be surprising if the men seldom, if ever, washed themselves, and may never have washed their clothes. The constant abrasion of dirty clothes on dirty, wet skin, and the scratching of hundreds of mosquito bites with filthy, work-worn fingernails must have rubbed bacteria into the skin. Boils and infections were an expected outcome.

Some historians have suggested that the boils were a manifestation of scurvy. Yet there is no evidence that the men of the Corps of Discovery ever had scurvy. The clinical signs of scurvy were described in graphic detail in 1602 by Father Antonio de la Ascension, a missionary exploring the coast of California.

> The first symptom they notice is a pain in the whole body which makes it sensitive to the touch . . . the body, especially from the waist down, becomes covered with purple spots larger than the great mustard seeds . . . the legs and the thighs become so straight and stiff . . . that they cannot be extended or drawn up . . . the teeth become so loose and without support that they move while moving the head . . . with this they cannot eat anything but food in liquid form or drinks . . . their natural vigor fails them and they die all of a sudden, while talking.

Scurvy develops after about a hundred days on a diet without vitamin C. At no time did the men of the Lewis and Clark expedition go that long without any green plants or fruit, and recent research has found buffalo meat to be particularly rich in vitamin C. According to journal records the men never exhibited anything like the horrific symptoms of incipient scurvy. Dental problems are not mentioned in the journals either (although Lewis took some dental instruments with him). The bleeding, the rashes, the devastating weakness and generalized body pains, and the failure of cuts to heal were not mentioned. Scurvy is a very improbable explanation for the boils and skin problems.

James Lind, a surgeon in the British Navy doing research on scurvy, performed a critical experiment in 1746. He studied a group of twelve scorbutic sailors, divided them into pairs, and tried six different treatments. The two sailors who received lemon and orange juice recovered quickly. The sailors who took either vinegar or sulfuric acid received no benefit. This experiment, one of the first "controlled studies," clearly pointed to the benefits of citrus fruits, but it was many years before ships routinely carried fruits and fresh vegetables to prevent scurvy. Benjamin Rush gave Lewis no advice about scurvy although it was a disease well known in America and common among some Indian tribes. Lewis and Clark were solicitous about the health of their men, but they seldom expressed any doubts about the nature of the diet they were eating, only about the lack of food at some times, and the dreariness and unpalatability of the food at others.

Boils were not the only problem, although they seemed to be the most common and most difficult to treat. Dysentery was also common and must have been related to poor camp hygiene and the drinking of foul river water. When the men began to take water from deeper in the river and not accept what was floating on the surface, many of their troubles ceased. One of the French engagés developed a serious chest infection that Clark had to lance. Sergeant Charles Floyd had a bad cold. Clark hurt his hand. Another of the engagés developed a large abscess in his thigh that had been present for about ten days before it was opened and began to bleed. Abscesses were opened when they became large and painful, the correct treatment for them as there were no antibiotics that could abort the infection before it became serious. Fortunately, the drainage of an abscess, even a large one, is often sufficient to cure it without antibiotics. Clark once awoke with a severe pain in the neck that he described as "rheumatism" and we might call "a crick in the neck." This painful but short-lived problem got better on its own.

Food was always on the men's minds as they strove westward. They were expending prodigious numbers of calories every day and, when well fed, were consuming more than 6,000 calories a day.

A modern dietitian would probably not approve of the diet. There was a preponderance of protein, very little fat, except what they obtained from the animal meat, only small amounts of carbohydrates, and variable quantities of fruit. If the diet might not now be regarded as "balanced" it might have met the approval of those who advocate a high-protein diet for losing weight, although weight loss would have been the last triviality on the men's minds. Later in the voyage, while they were going through the Rockies, their diet was marginal and the efforts they spent were great. Added to this, they had an epidemic of diarrhea, and all of the men must have lost weight. But, in the first phase of the journey, ascending the Missouri to the land of the Mandans, lack of food was not a problem.

The intent had always been to live off the land, supplementing what they killed with the flour, cereals, and salt pork they brought with them. It would have been impossible to bring sufficient provisions to feed forty-five men for months on end. Almost every day the journals detailed the number of deer, elk, and other animals killed for food or scientific collection. Two deer and a bear. Five deer and a bear. One fat bear and a deer. Eleven deer and a wolf. A badger. Pronghorn antelope. Bighorn sheep. Later, when the Corps reached the land of the buffalo, the herds were a walking larder, there for the picking. They also caught and ate beaver, porcupine, elk, and, later in the voyage, many dogs and horses. Whatever was available and edible.

Not everyone always ate his fill. George Shannon, the youngest member of the Corps became separated from the group and spent two weeks by himself in a desperate search for the boats. During that time he ate berries and one rabbit, which he killed with a stick shot from his rifle. When he finally caught up, he was near the end of his endurance. Although hunters for the group frequently went away in pairs or small groups, this escapade was the only time one man became lost and isolated. He may have been in desperate straits when he finally rejoined the others, but he never gave up. At least he had the river to guide him and never encountered hostile Indians. Being lost and separated from friends, even for a day or two, is the true test of an outdoorsman, and it is to the credit of this nineteen-year-old man that he kept his cool and survived. (Many years later he lost a leg in a battle with the Indians along the Missouri, left the Army and became a lawyer.)

The Missouri River valley's land was rich in fruit, and the diet of meat was lightened with gooseberries, cherries, raspberries, grapes, and red and black currants. The men collected "greens" along the banks of the river, and Clark recorded sending York, his servant, to pick cress for their meal. Fish were plentiful and, in one place, they were able to net more than eight hundred fish in a day—perch, pike, and catfish. Gass recorded catching nine catfish, which together weighed 300 pounds, with hook and line. Lewis wrote that they never killed more than they needed for their immediate needs, although, later in the voyage, they sometimes shot elk purely to get hides for clothing or boats and left the meat to rot. If they had excess meat they dried and smoked it to make jerky, the best way of preserving it, and good for eating when the hunters could not supply all they needed.

June 18, 1804, was spent off the river, and the men were put to work making and repairing ropes and oars. The hunters killed five deer and Colter shot a very fat bear. It rained all day, and, in spite of this, the men tried to dry meat and they greased their own skin (perhaps as a protection against mosquito bites). Several men had dysentery and two-thirds of them had boils or ulcers, some with eight or ten boils. The mosquitoes were very bad. It was enough to make a reasonable man long for the comforts of home, but the final journal entry for the day was "Men in spirits."

Independence Day was ushered in with a blast from the blunderbuss on the bow of the keelboat. Then, when the men went ashore, Joseph Fields was bitten on the foot by a rattlesnake. Captain Lewis doctored the bite with a poultice of Peruvian bark, a common cure for snakebites to which gunpowder was sometimes added. With a very bad bite the gunpowder might be set alight. That Fields' foot became swollen indicated that the bite was not "dry." Some venom was injected, but the snake was most likely a small prairie rattler without seriously destructive venom.

Rattlesnake venom causes severe pain, and one of the ways to determine whether a snake has injected venom is to ask about pain. If there is no pain shortly after the bite, the snake probably did not inject venom. A dose of laudanum or opium would have made Fields more comfortable. Ordway, Floyd, and Gass all mentioned in their diaries that Fields was bitten. Floyd remarked that the foot became badly swollen, and Gass added, "but not dangerously." The incident was not worth mentioning again the next day. Poor Fields presumably limped for a couple of days but did not receive much sympathy.

There are four species of venomous snakes in the United States: rattlesnakes, copperheads, water moccasins, and coral snakes. Only rattlesnakes would have been encountered along the route of the expedition. There are many subspecies of rattlesnakes, but the two most likely to be met were the prairie rattler (*Crotalus viridis*) and, later on the trip, the Pacific rattler (*Crotalus viridis oreganus*). The large and dangerous diamondback rattlers do not live as far north, which was just as well. The encounters the men had with snakes were relatively benign. They saw many snakes, sometimes frighteningly close, but only two men were bitten and neither suffered severe complications.

Rattlesnake venom causes necrosis of tissue, and the amount of damage depends—as was rightly conjectured by Lewis' advisor Benjamin Barton—on the species of snake, its size, and the volume of venom injected. Some bites, such as the one suffered by Fields, cause swelling and pain for a few days. Others result in swelling, pain, blistering of the skin, and black-and-bloody gangrene and loss of fingers, toes, hands, and feet. It was fortunate that the expedition was traveling by boat and Fields could continue with his duties. If they had been on foot, gangrene would have been a disaster, and even a relatively mild bite, such as he had, would have prevented him from marching. As antivenin is the only effective treatment for a severe bite, the absence of treatment would have doomed anyone with severe complications to death or disablement.

As the expedition ventured on, other issues abounded. Discipline, which had been a problem at the Wood River Camp, continued to be a problem as they progressed up the Missouri. Collins and Hall were charged with getting drunk by tapping the whiskey supply they were supposed to guard. Collins pled not guilty, but was sentenced to one hundred lashes on his bare back. Hall received fifty lashes.

Alexander Hamilton Willard, who had also been in trouble at St. Charles, was later found asleep while on guard, a much more serious offense than drunkenness, and punishable by death. The expedition was in country where the friendliness of the Indians was in doubt. A sneak night attack would have been both possible and likely. In all armies, for a sentry to sleep while on guard or to leave a position is a grave offense, liable to the most severe punishment. Willard pled guilty to lying down but did not plead guilty to being asleep. He was sentenced to one hundred lashes, to be delivered twenty-five lashes at a time, on four successive evenings.

The disciplinary troubles were not over. A month later, on August 4, Moses Reed and one of the French boatmen were sent back to a previous camp to collect a knife that had been left behind, and they did not return on time. Reed may have left his knife behind as an excuse to go back to "find" it. Clark believed that Reed had deserted. On August 6, Clark sent back four men to find and capture Reed, dead or alive, and to look for, but not necessarily kill, the Frenchman who was not subject to the same military laws. The search party included the incomparable, reliable George Drewyer. More than a week later, on August 17, the search party returned with Reed but without the Frenchman who had been recaptured and then escaped.

Reed was tried and was probably lucky to escape with his life. The court condemned him to run four times through a gantlet of the men of the Corps who thrashed his back with their ramrods as he ran. He received about five hundred lashes and was denied the chance of remaining as a permanent member of the Corps that would go to the West Coast.

Two months passed without another severe disciplinary problem. But in mid-October John Newman was confined for mutinous expressions. He was tried and sentenced to seventy-five lashes and, like Reed, was discharged from the expedition. The court was not

unanimous in its verdict; one-third of the nine-man court dis-
agreed. Newman was, nonetheless, punished and was additionally
condemned to labor as a hand on one of the pirogues. Instead of
doing guard duty he was to become a general pariah, being given
"such drudgeries as they may think proper to direct from time to
time with a view to the general relief of the detachment." Fancy
language, which gave license to the rest of the group to assign
Newman every stinking job they could think of.

Newman's flogging caused great distress to a visiting Indian
Chief who said that they never whipped their people, even from the
youngest age. When Clark explained the nature of the crime and
the system of justice the Chief was mollified and agreed that he had
sometimes had to order the execution of his own people. Newman
did everything he could to reinstate himself in the good graces of
his officers and must have accepted every "drudgery" imposed on
him with goodwill. But Lewis would not relent, and when the time
came to send some of the group back to Washington after the winter was over, Newman had to leave. Years later, however, Lewis did
recommend to the President that Newman be rewarded for his
faithful service, but he paid a heavy price for a few ill-considered,
angry words.

Nothing is said in the journals about the wounds inflicted by
flogging, nor about any treatment given or how the injuries
affected the ability of the men to work. It is hard to believe that
Willard, who was flogged every evening for four nights, could have
pulled his weight working on the boat with a bleeding, swollen
back on which the touch of a shirt would have been agony. The
mosquitoes were beginning to become an intolerable pest, and a
bleeding back covered with mosquitoes and deer flies must have
been worse punishment than the actual flogging. The diaries of
Ordway and others make little mention of the trials and the punishments. Perhaps they were so inured to the standards and methods of
discipline that a flogging was not worthy of comment.

Newman's trial was the last. During, and after, the winter in Fort
Mandan the morale of the group coalesced and they were moti-

vated by a single-minded drive to get the job done. Success became a matter of pride. And, as in all well-led, elite military units, hardship, challenge, and apparently insuperable difficulties increase, rather than decrease morale, thereby solidifying the esprit de corps.

As soon as the weather became warm, mosquitoes and ticks became a pest, especially the mosquitoes. Lewis had brought mosquito netting for himself and the men to sleep under, and this must have relieved them at night. There were tents among the supplies, but there is not a good description of how the camps were set up or how the mosquito netting was used. Later, when the netting had been torn and used a hundred times, there were complaints about the mosquitoes, and one night when Lewis was away from the river and forgot his netting, he paid the price of his forgetfulness with a very uncomfortable night.

Mosquitoes are most abundant at dawn and dusk, but on the boats in the river, with a good breeze blowing, they would not have been a problem. But no matter where the group made camp on shore, if there was not a strong wind the mosquitoes would have been unbearable. There is no evidence from the record of the Corps' sicknesses that they suffered from mosquito-borne diseases. There was an occasional reference to "ague" which might or might not have been malaria. But there are no descriptions of full-blown malaria with attacks of fever every three or four days, and violent shivering followed by profuse sweating. No one developed encephalitis, another mosquito-borne disease that frequently occurs, even now, in small epidemics along the Mississippi and Missouri Rivers.

Meanwhile, Lewis seemed to keep healthier than Clark, but when Lewis became sick, he became quite sick. At the end of August 1804, during one of those periods when Lewis was writing very little in his journal, he suffered a self-inflicted episode that could have been very serious. Some of the men, including Lewis, went ashore at a bluff that contained numerous minerals—copperas, cobalt, pyrites, and others. Lewis tasted some of the minerals, smelled the rocks, and became sick. "Capt. Lewis in proveing the quality of those minerals was near poisoning himself by the fumes and taste of the cobalt which had the appearance of soft isonglass [a form of gelatin]." Later in the day Lewis took a dose of salts to work off the effects of arsenic and cobalt. It is not clear exactly what he took, and the reference to arsenic is obscure. There was a rumor that Black Bird, a prominent local Indian Chief, had been in the habit of poisoning his enemies and rivals with arsenic obtained from the banks of the river. Clark recorded how ill-tasting the waters of the river were and how they were responsible for illness among the men. As there was no chemical analysis of what Lewis tasted or drank it is impossible to guess at the toxicity of the minerals or the river.

In addition to mosquitoes and ticks, and injuries from everyday labors, the climate and the elements greatly affected the health of the men at all times, whether in summer or winter. On July 7, 1804, the morning temperature was 96°F (35.6°C) and probably very humid. One of the men, Robert Frazier, became very sick "struck by the sun" and was treated by Lewis with a dose of niter and by being bled, which apparently relieved his symptoms. The next day several men were sick with violent headaches, also perhaps related to working in the sun.

Heat illness affects the body in several different ways, but the basic problem is always the same. The body produces more heat than it can dissipate and overheats. Body temperature is a constant balance between heat production and retention against heat loss and gain. Muscles and internal organs produce heat, and several mechanisms, of which sweating is the most important, help dissipate excess body heat. In a very hot environment the body absorbs heat from the sun while also producing its own metabolic heat. A center in the brain that controls body temperature recognizes when the body is overheating and initiates mechanisms for losing heat. Sweating helps dissipate heat by evaporation from the skin, (530 kilocalorie/liter sweat evaporated), and the small vessels of the skin dilate, increasing heat loss to the surrounding environment. If the atmosphere is very humid, as it is in many parts of the United States during the summer and as it probably was on that day in

1804, sweating is an inefficient method for losing heat because the moisture in the air is in balance with the moisture on the skin. Sweating occurs, but there is little evaporation. It is evaporation that cools, not the sweating. In a very hot, dry climate sweating is very efficient because evaporation is rapid and the body cools.

There are several types of heat illness, including heat exhaustion, heat cramps, and heatstroke. In heat exhaustion, which was probably the problem with Frazier, there is excessive loss of fluid and electrolytes in the sweat. The person becomes dehydrated, and may faint or become extremely tired because of a fall in blood pressure. The current treatment is to remove the victim from the heat and provide large volumes of fluids containing the appropriate electrolytes. If there is an excessive loss of sodium and potassium the muscles cramp and the person doubles up in pain. Fluids and electrolytes are again the cure, and stretching the muscles relieves the pain. Heatstroke is the most critical form of heat illness, and can be fatal. If the body is producing a lot of heat because of exertion, while absorbing heat from a strong sun, sweating and evaporation may be inadequate to reduce the body temperature, which rises dramatically. The body temperature may rise as high as 106°F (41°C). A temperature of 108°F (42.2°C) is fatal. The victim collapses, becomes unconscious, and may have convulsions because of the effect of the high body temperature on the brain. As an authority on heat illness has said, "It does not take long to boil an egg or to cook neurons."

Heatstroke is a medical emergency requiring rapid cooling of the body in addition to restoration of fluids and electrolytes. We do not know Frazier's temperature but can say with confidence that he did not have heatstroke. He did not become unconscious or have serious neurological complications, and he survived. Bleeding would have been disastrous treatment for heatstroke, and equally bad for heat exhaustion. Niter induces a profound sweat and was used to reduce fevers. Paradoxically, it may have done some good by making Frazier sweat even more and increase heat loss. The best treatment would have been to put him in the shade with lots of water to drink and a piece of salt pork to chew. A dip in the river would have done no harm. Once again, good luck rather than good management intervened, and Frazier survived.

President Jefferson had enjoined Lewis to avoid conflict with the Indians, if at all possible, and the expedition followed his orders as it continued up the Missouri. The reactions of most of the tribes could be foretold because traders had been traveling the lower stretches of the Missouri for many years and were familiar with the Indians. One tribe, however, was a cause for genuine worry: the Sioux. This was the largest, most powerful, most warlike tribe of the plains. For many years they had been stopping traders as they went along the river and extracting from them a steady toll of furs and supplies. The Yankton Sioux, the first branch of the tribe that Lewis and Clark met, were friendly, and there were no problems as they passed through the Yankton Territory. The Teton Sioux were different.

What did Lewis really understand about the Indians he would meet? He had been acquainted with the forest Indians of the East, but he probably knew little about the culture or history of the Plains Indians. His approach to all the tribes was the same. A meeting was called with the Chiefs, there was an exchange of gifts, a pipe was smoked, a meal was eaten, and speeches were made. Then there was a show of military drill and the firepower of the Corps. Interpretation of the speeches was a problem, and the subtleties of meaning passing from one side to the other were often missed. Lewis had a standard stump speech, somewhat like a modern politician seeking office. The Indians, addressed as "Children," were told of the Great White Father in Washington, his huge power, but his intention to keep the peace as long as the Indians behaved and kept their side of the bargain. The tribes were urged not to fight their neighbors. In return traders would come and bring the goods the Indians needed and wanted.

In retrospect, Lewis' speeches were patronizing and ignorant of Indian politics. They wanted whiskey and guns, the goods the French and British had been trading for furs. They were not always happy with medals and fancy speeches. In spite of these failings, and because most of the Indians wanted to be at peace with the white men, the expedition was successful in staying out of trouble. One of Lewis' repeated themes was that the white man was to be trusted, a theme that subsequent history proved disastrously untrue. A major battle with Indians would have been a catastrophe and the end of the expedition. The Corps was well armed and did not fail to demonstrate its strength. It was probably a combination of this display of power and patience in negotiating that prevented any major showdown.

If there had been a battle with the Indians, and even if the Corps had been victorious, their medical supplies—including one small set of surgical instruments—were totally inadequate to deal with the number of arrow and gunshot wounds they would have sustained. The fifty dozen Rush's Thunderbolts in their medical chest would have been no help. The death toll would have been terrible. If anyone had survived, a retreat downstream would have been a journey of horror. They would have been attacked from the riverbanks day and night, while trying to defend themselves and deal with their wounded at the same time. Lady Luck was on their side again.

One aspect of Indian culture that was not displeasing to the Corps was their habit of offering women to visiting men. Even the warlike Sioux tried to use women in their diplomatic negotiations. In the Brulé village Lewis and Clark were offered companions for their beds. Clark wrote that "there is a curious custom with the Sioux as well as the rickerres [the Arikaras] is to give handsom squars to those whome they wish to show some acknowledgements to." The Captains, in what may have been a diplomatic faux pas, declined the offer. It may not have been a polite move to refuse the offer, but it might have been a sensible one. Venereal disease was common among the Indians, and the men of the Corps who took advantage of the hospitality often ended up with unpleasant consequences. The Indians regarded sexual intercourse not just as physical pleasure but as a means of transferring spiritual strength from the man to the woman. If the visitor was an important man, then the strength of the spiritual transfer was even greater. The power of the visitor was passed to the woman and then back to the woman's husband. Women were very important in these societies, but their lives were hard, planting and raising crops, caring for the children, making the clothes, gathering firewood, and cooking while the men hunted, fought wars, and defended their people. The men did not always treat their wives well but still recognized their importance to the community.

The Sioux were nomadic, following the bison herds, but the Arikaras, who lived upstream, were the agriculturists of the plains, growing large crops of corn, beans, tobacco, and other produce. The women tilled the fields with diggers made from the shoulder blades of buffalo and deer—hard work that Lewis and Clark regarded as further evidence of the drudgery that was the lot of women. The tribe lived in permanent villages, and it was in those villages that the men of the expedition later experienced the sexual liberality they found so attractive. Clark's black servant York was a particular favorite and a source of wonder and fear. The Indians could not believe that his skin was not painted, but his size and mock fearsome behavior scared some of them who believed that he ate children. He was especially attractive to the women who thought that to have sex with him would endow them with special powers. York apparently did nothing to dissuade the women of that opinion, and there were later, unsubstantiated, reports of curly-headed children among the Arikaras.

Smallpox decimated the Arikaras in 1780, and again a couple of years before the Lewis and Clark expedition passed through their land. The Corps saw deserted villages and heard from the Indians of the terror and destruction the disease had brought to them. Once again good fortune was on the side of the expedition. If they had mingled with the Arikaras in the middle of the smallpox epidemic many of the men would undoubtedly have become infected, and the expedition would have come to an end. After leaving the Arikaras in October the expedition entered the land of the Hidatsas and Mandans where the men would spend the long winter months of 1804–1805 among friendly people from whom they would learn much about the journey ahead.

On July 31, 1804, Sergeant Floyd recorded in his diary that he had been very sick but had recovered. On August 19, the Sergeant suddenly fell desperately ill. Within twenty-four hours he was dead. This crisis has reverberated down through the years. The cause of his death has been the subject of prolonged discussion, without the possibility of resolution. Sergeant Floyd was the first U.S soldier to die west of the Mississippi and the only member of the Corps to die. His friends buried him with military honors on a hill beside the river and placed a cedar marker over his grave. As the men marched down from the hill, back to the river and the tasks of the moment, they must have looked at themselves and the men beside them and wondered who might be the next to die. They knew they had embarked on a long and dangerous journey. They had fought in wars and lived in a tough and hazardous environment. They were no strangers to death.

For a modern medical detective or physician there are frustrating gaps in the evidence regarding Floyd's condition. We can deduce that he suffered from either two separate illnesses or two bouts of the same illness. We know that the second episode was catastrophic and killed Floyd in twenty-four hours. We also know that during his final hours he was vomiting, experiencing severe diarrhea, and rapidly developed shock with a barely palpable pulse.

The basic requirements for making a diagnosis of an illness such as Floyd's are a good history and a physical examination. The descriptions of Floyd's illness are graphic but skimpy, and unfortunately there was no physical examination. Vomiting and diarrhea are often symptoms of an abdominal illness, and the combination of sudden, uncontrollable vomiting and diarrhea excludes almost every diagnosis other than an abdominal problem.

Were the two illnesses connected or not? On July 31, Floyd indicated "I am verry sick and has ben for Somtime but have recovered my health again." Lewis only described that Floyd was "verry unwell" and had a "bad Cold &c." The evidence would suggest that the illness in July was respiratory. If Floyd had a respiratory infection at the end of July, then there is no likely connection between it and his subsequent death. If he had an intestinal problem in July, it would be reasonable to connect the two episodes.

Without the results of a physical examination during the final illness, making a diagnosis is pure speculation. Physical examination of patients was not an integral part of diagnosis in 1800, and Clark, who had no medical training, cannot be blamed for failing to slip a hand under Floyd's shirt to feel his belly. Even a doctor of that day might not have made a physical examination. The question is, what was going on inside his abdomen?

For many years a theory has been passed from book to book, that Floyd died from a ruptured appendix. Bernard De Voto, who was a wonderful historian, but not a doctor, wrote that Floyd suffered an attack of appendicitis in late July and that his appendix ruptured three weeks later. This is possible, but very unlikely. Between July 31 and August 20, Floyd had been performing his full share of duties on the boat, and there was no suggestion in his own journal of abdominal pain, feeling sick, or being unable to perform his responsibilities. On August 8, he had walked for miles along the shore with Clark and had even gone on a fishing expedition with several of the men during which they caught more than three hundred fish. These are not the activities of a man with an appendiceal abscess grumbling away in his abdomen for three weeks. Floyd would surely have made some remark in his journal about a continuing problem with his health. Yet, he declared himself as having recovered and being in good health on July 30 and never mentioned another problem.

The appendix, a wormlike appendage, hangs off the lower end of the cecum, the first part of the large intestine on the right side of the abdomen. Because it is a cul-de-sac, it may become clogged by anything from a small concretion of feces to a fruit seed. When this happens, the contents between the obstruction and the tip of the appendix fester, and the organ becomes inflamed. The inflamed appendix rubs against the inside of the abdominal muscles and causes pain. The sufferer gets cramplike upper abdominal pain, usually vomits, develops a mild fever, loses all appetite, and tends to want to lie still because movement increases the pain—but rarely has diarrhea. Over the course of several hours or a day the pain settles in the lower right side of the abdomen. If the infection is virulent, it may weaken the wall of the appendix, causing the organ to rupture. Rupture is rarely a spontaneous, explosive event, but rather starts with a slow leak and the development of an abscess around the appendix over a couple of days. Sometimes the infection spreads throughout the entire abdominal cavity with the development of peritonitis (an inflammation of the abdominal cavity lining), a potentially catastrophic illness. This, however, is a process that takes time, and, in its early stages, the patient is very uncomfortable, obviously very sick, but not about to die within hours.

Something quick and disastrous happened to Sergeant Floyd. He was well one morning and then, the next morning, he was "taken verry bad all at once." The critical words in Clark's observations are "all at once." There are few infections or illnesses that develop "all at once." Sudden physiological changes, such as a stroke or heart attack, are often vascular; and most, but not all, infections take at least a day to develop. The rupture of an organ can be sudden; but the perforation of an infected appendix is a slower, less dramatic affair. Floyd's illness not only started instantaneously, but it also proceeded to induce shock and death within twenty-four hours.

Possibilities, other than appendicitis, that might have caused Floyd's sudden death include a perforated duodenal ulcer, a ruptured aneurysm, an obstructed blood supply to his gut, or an overwhelming intestinal infection caused by a very potent organism. There are pros and cons for each of these diagnoses. Floyd was young, making a ruptured aortic aneurysm unlikely. The blockage of the blood supply to Floyd's intestine is possible, but again, unlikely. Rupture of a duodenal ulcer would not have killed him as rapidly.

In the opinions of several distinguished abdominal surgeons, there are too many contradictory clues—the sudden onset of shock, the profuse diarrhea combined with vomiting, the absence of a clear premonitory phase—to be able to say pontifically, "Floyd died from appendicitis." The combination of vomiting and diarrhea leading to shock is almost unknown in a "surgical" abdominal catastrophe. These symptoms are quite possible with an overwhelming intestinal infection, but it is difficult to say what the infectious organism might have been. As of 1800, cholera had not appeared in North America. A perforated typhoid ulcer of the intestine might have been possible. Other organisms, such as *campylobacter*, or some strains of *E. Coli*, now recognized as a cause of catastrophic intestinal infections, could also have produced such an emergency. These organisms, however, have only recently been recognized as causes of death.

While historians continue to suggest a ruptured appendix as the cause of Floyd's death, the recorded symptoms as well as recent medical evaluations of the evidence in the journals, put more weight on the diagnosis of a severe and lethal infection. Although the death of Sergeant Floyd made no difference to the ultimate achievements of the expedition, it was a terrible psychological blow to the Corps of Discovery. He did not go down in a blaze of glory fighting Indians, but rather, died from a quick, unexpected disease. Those who were left did not know what had happened. Some of them must have wondered if this mysterious illness could strike them next. The men were used to death and disease, but the sudden death of a young friend, without an explanation, raised the most disturbing fears and questions.

Two days later Patrick Gass was elected to fill the place of Floyd as Sergeant. The ranks had closed. Later, on the return home, some of the men went to Floyd's grave, but the visit was brief. Too much had happened in the intervening years. The pain of his death had passed.

FIVE

Winter with the Mandans:
November 1804–March 1805

In 1742 Le Chevalier and Francois Vérendryes ventured south from Fort La Reine on the Assiniboine River to "that civilized white nation living to the west of this country on the shore of the sea." The two men left the sheltering woods around their fort in October and marched across the plains, not sure of what they would find. In December of the same year, they entered a Mandan village along the Missouri River, a town of 150 houses surrounded with fortifications. The inhabitants were light-skinned, but they were, without doubt, Indians. During the following four years Le Chevalier and Francois traveled through the Mandan country in a wide sweep to the south and west, returning up the Missouri, with reports of a river that headed west and ended in the ocean.

In the nearly one hundred years before Lewis and Clark arrived in the Missouri River valley, the British and French had traded continuously with the Mandans who were known to be peaceful and honest. The Mandans were the middlemen for the trade between the whites of the Northeast and the Plains tribes that sought guns, whiskey, powder, knives, pots, needles, awls, and fishhooks.

The expedition, therefore, was not arriving in unexplored territory. This, of course, was one of the reasons Lewis and Clark chose to spend the winter among the Mandans. They had already had many contacts with whites and had proved themselves to be useful partners in trade. When the Corps of Discovery arrived at the Mandan village on October 27, 1804, they found a British trader,

Hugh McCracken, who had arrived a few days before, and a Frenchman, René Jessaume, who had lived with the Mandans for about thirteen years. Both men were evidence of the continuing threat to American trade by the British and French, and Lewis made it clear that authority over the land had changed and the traders must not sell or distribute flags or medals that would promote their countries.

The first job, after making initial contact with the local Chief, was to search for a place where the Corps could build their winter quarters. They needed to find a place close enough to the Mandan village for easy contact, but not so close that the Corps would be troubled by a constant stream of visitors. There were at least five large Mandan and Hidatsa villages in the area, some housing hundreds of warriors and their families. The Corps also needed to find a spot with plenty of large cottonwood trees for logs to build a fort. They eventually settled on a site downstream from the two main Mandan villages, on the east bank of the river, where the wood was good and game was abundant.

After spending a fruitless day searching for the right place Clark returned to their temporary camp and found many visiting Indians to whom he gave whiskey. Then everyone had a dance, presumably with Cruzatte doing the musical honors. More ceremonies that day interrupted Clark's search for a winter campsite. The main Chief of one the Mandan villages invited Clark to an elaborate gathering where "with great ceremony I was seated on a robe by the side of the Chief." The Chief promised peace and blamed recent fighting on another Chief and some hot-blooded young men. He returned two traps that had been stolen from the French engagés and gave Clark two bushels of corn. The Chief visited the camp again that night dressed in a new suit he had been given and everyone danced until 10:00.

The Mandans were genuinely pleased to have the expedition in the area. It provided political security and freedom from war, at least as long as they were there. The Chief said that "peace not only gives me pleasure, but the satisfaction to all the nation. They now can hunt without fear, and our womin can work in the fields without looking every moment for the enimey."

Winter was approaching fast. The winds were increasing in force, and there was a threat of ice on the river. On November 1, before they rowed to their winter campsite, the wind blew so hard that the men were unable to work until the evening when the storm stopped. Then the boats were able to drop 7 miles downstream to the wooded site that Clark had found. The next day, Clark set the men to work cutting down trees. Hunting for food was still an essential task, and Clark sent out hunters every day looking for deer, beaver, buffalo, and elk. As the weeks went by and deer became more scarce the men sometimes had to eat meat, such as wolves, that they would normally have refused.

On November 4, a Frenchman named Touissaint Charbonneau appeared at camp with his two wives, one of whom was called Sacagawea. Both were Shoshone (Snake) Indians from the Rockies. Charbonneau could interpret various Indian languages, so Lewis immediately engaged him to join the expedition. Sacagawea would come to interpret the Shoshone language, although the Corps was many months away from entering their land. Lewis saw this as a providential chance to have a native interpreter who could negotiate with a tribe that was most important to them. The Shoshones had horses, and the friendly acquisition of horses from them was essential to a successful crossing of the Shining Mountains, as the Indians called the Rockies.

In the midst of all this activity Clark had a bad attack of rheumatism; perhaps a return of the "crick in the neck" of which he had complained earlier. In spite of this, the building of the camp, which was to become known as Fort Mandan, went forward. When the fort was finally finished it was a considerable structure with a triangular base, 18-foot outer walls, and inner roofs that sloped down to a central open space used for mustering the troops. The houses were divided into living and storage quarters. A large swinging gate, also 18 feet tall, gave access to the fort. The Corps had no intention of being taken by surprise and, also, they wanted a fort that would be reasonably secure from wandering, inquisitive Indians who might want to come and spend the night trading, drinking, and dancing. The Captains knew that not all the Indian visitors would be men.

The Indians continued to visit in large numbers, and the arrival of the Corps was obviously the hit of the season. The Indians told the Corps that they had chosen a good site with wood and water, and that the bark of the cottonwood trees would provide excellent food for their horses in the winter. The Indians brought their own dogs and horses into their houses during the winter nights, in part to protect them from the bitter winter gales, but also to keep them from being stolen. In the summer they fed the horses on grass, but in the winter they fed them cottonwood bark. Later in the winter when Lewis tried to give some of the horses an extra treat by feeding them corn, they would not eat it and only ate cottonwood bark.

On November 10, Clark wrote, "The day raw and cold wind from the NW, the Gees continue to pass in gangues as also brant to the south, some ducks also pass." Two of the men cut themselves with axes while working on the fort, and Charbonneau's two Shoshone wives appeared for the first time at the camp. Charbonneau had bought his two wives from the Hidatsas who had in turn captured the women in a raid against the Snakes some years before and brought them across the plains to the Mandan area. The two women were around eleven or twelve years old when caught and were probably marched, terrified for their lives, across the plains while the men who had killed their relatives laughed and sang war songs of triumph. For the Hidatsas it had been a successful skirmish. Some of their young braves had gained honor; they had captured horses and were headed home with two young slaves who would become submissive wives to a brave. We know nothing of their long overland journey from the Rockies to the Missouri and the subsequent years during which the two girls lived with the Hidatsas.

What route did they take? What landmarks did the young girls imprint on their minds? Did they ever hope to escape or did they accept their imprisonment and slavery as part of Indian life? Perhaps they thought the best solution was to accept what fate had dealt them. Slavery had been a part of Indian life for centuries, and the two girls would have known that, having been captured, they would be slaves and wives. When Charbonneau joined the Corps the younger wife, Sacagawea, was pregnant, and the older one already had a small child.

Lewis' decision to take Charbonneau and one of the wives (there does not seem to have ever been an agreement to take both wives), was obviously logical. But who decided to take Sacagawea instead of the other wife? And why would the leader of an expedition want to take an Indian girl of about sixteen or seventeen, who would be carrying a newborn infant by the time the expedition started again in the spring? Charbonneau's other wife already had a child who was about two years old, and perhaps Lewis thought it would be easier to have a child that would be carried on its mother's back for most of the trip, rather than have a toddler running around the camp and disrupting life on the boats.

How many trip leaders, faced with a journey of several thousand miles, replete with unknown difficulties and hazards, would ever take along a sixteen-year-old girl with a newborn baby strapped to her back? Did Lewis, who at times had a rather impersonal attitude toward the Indians, assume that, because she was an Indian, she would be able to look after herself and that all would be well? Later in the trip when Sacagawea was very sick, and her life in doubt, Lewis did express concern for her as a person, but could not help coupling his concern for her with worry that they would lose a vital interpreter if she died.

By the middle of November the ice was beginning to flow on the river, and the men moved into their huts, and finally unloaded the boats before they became trapped in river ice for the winter. Two days after the men moved into the huts snow began to fall. The ice on the river became thicker. The cold hand of winter was closing around them. The temperature fell, and fell, and fell until it reached its lowest reading of –74°F (-58° C). The men went hunting in an icy mist, and the temperature became so cold that the sentries had to be relieved every half hour.

The hunters returned on November 19 with thirty-two deer, twelve elk, and a buffalo. All the meat was hung in the smokehouse they had built, a timely supply. Because of the huge amounts of meat the men ate every day—up to 9 pounds per man on some days—even a generous supply had to be continuously renewed. They supplemented their diet with corn they received in trade, and as gifts, from the Indians. Corn, exchanged for metalwork, was the most popular form of trade. The blacksmith fired up his forge and made axes, tomahawks, and farming tools. These were the tools the Indians normally bought from the visiting British and French, and they were delighted to have their weapons custom-made for them by the smith. A local Chief thought the blacksmith was the most useful member of the expedition. Lewis thought the design of the Indians' battle-ax was inefficient, but no one was about to change it when the trade brought in a steady supply of corn. That probably supplied more carbohydrates than they had had in their diet for some time. As a producer of energy and maintainer of body fat the corn was very useful and would continue to be a staple throughout the winter.

The energy requirements of the men were just as great during this period as when they were rowing and pulling up the river. Cold imposes a huge demand on the body for energy to maintain body heat. In addition, the men were sometimes exerting themselves to exhaustion. The hunting trips frequently took them up to 50 miles away from the camp. Then, if they were successful, they had to drag the meat back to the fort on crude sleds. On one occasion sixteen men were required to drag the sleds 21 miles back to the fort over hard ice and snow. Their feet were cold, painful, and near to frostbite. The skin on their cheeks was nipped by the frost. They needed all they could eat and should have had more fat in their diet. Protein and carbohydrates each produce 4 calories per gram, but fat produces 9 calories per gram. The fat in meat allowed the men to get more energy from an ounce of meat than they could from an ounce of corn. The men of the modern U.S. Army, living and exercising in a cold climate such as Alaska, eat a 4,000 to 5,000 calorie diet every day.

Relations with the Indians were, on the whole, good. During the winter there were many visitors from numerous tribes—Mandans, Hidatsas, Arikaras, Cheyenne, Gros Ventres, and even another pair of Snake Indians who were probably slaves caught, like Sacagawea, in a raid. If the visitor was a Chief he would be presented with medals, clothes, tobacco, and entertained in the fort. Occasionally an important visitor was invited to sleep overnight in the fort, although this was not encouraged. Sometimes the crowds were big, and Ordway once recorded that he had fourteen Indians eating in his cabin at one time. On Christmas day, 1804, the men requested that there be no visitors, as this day was "big medicine." The Indians respected the request, and the men were able to celebrate Christmas with extra food, drink, and dancing.

Dancing was popular with the men of the Corps and the Indians. Sometimes the men would go to the Mandan village and move from hut to hut dancing and "frolicking." One of the Frenchmen, François Rivet, could dance on his head. Break dancing on the Missouri! These evenings often ended with some of the men staying in the Indians' huts, presumably with a friendly companion, although not all the Indians were happy about their wives having relations with the soldiers.

Early in January 1805, the Mandans carried out a traditional ceremony to attract the returning buffalo. They held a three-night dance that included what Clark described as a "curious custom" The old men sat in a circle and the young men came in with their wives, who were dressed only in a single robe. The young men approached the old men in a "whining tone" and asked them to accept their wives and sleep with them. The old men disappeared with the women for sexual intercourse. If an old man—for whatever reason—could not complete his part of the compact, the young man would entreat him repeatedly not to refuse the offer. This ceremony was based on two beliefs: first, that intercourse would pass the hunting skills and experience of the old man to the woman, and then to the young man. Second, it was hoped that the ceremony would attract more buffalo to the hunt. Visiting men were particularly attractive recipients of the favors offered by the husbands, and they did not hesitate to participate.

Venereal disease was a continuing and serious complication of these alliances. The Captains did not make clear how many of their men developed venereal disease, but Clark's comments in his journal that one man was "very bad with the pox" and later, that the men "were generally healthy except Venerial complaints which is verry common amongst the natives and the men catch it from them," indicated that venereal disease was common. Clark did not acknowledge that the men were also responsible for spreading the disease. Any man with either syphilis or gonorrhea who continued to consort with the women was likely, at some moment, to spread what he had to an uninfected woman. Sexually transmitted diseases travel on a two-way street.

The most common form of treatment for venereal diseases in the nineteenth century was mercury used either as a salve on the genital sores, or given as a pill in the form of calomel. Treatment was continued until excessive salivation, an early sign of mercury poisoning, became obvious. Lewis brought adequate supplies of mercury in the medical kit, obviously anticipating the problems. There were also penis syringes in the surgical kit for irrigating the urethra of infected men. As nothing was known about sterilization of instruments one shudders to think how the use of the syringes could also have spread the diseases.

The men, living in Fort Mandan in close quarters, began to get colds, and John Shields developed rheumatism, a complaint that is mentioned many times without a clear definition of the symptoms. As it never appeared to be permanent, with swelling of the joints and continuing disability, the term was probably used to describe general aching joints, back pain, and other musculoskeletal problems. A more obvious joint problem occurred when Sergeant Nathaniel Pryor was taking down the mast of the keelboat and dislocated his shoulder. As the mast was 32 feet high, it is easy to understand that if it suddenly fell backward, pulling the Sergeant's arm, a dislocation could happen. Four attempts were necessary to reduce the shoulder. The usual method at that time for reducing a dislocated shoulder had been described by Hippocrates. The victim was first laid on his or her back. The manipulator then put a foot in the injured person's armpit while, at the same time, pulling strongly on the affected arm. The purpose of the foot was to provide counterpressure against the chest while there was a strong pull on the arm. The method works as well now as when it was described by Hippocrates, but it has the danger of fracturing the top end of the humerus while reducing the dislocation. And if the humerus is already fractured—a not uncommon concomitant complication—the situation can be made worse rather than better. Sergeant Pryor, however, returned to duty without any complications.

Daily life at the fort continued with hunting, visiting, repairing of clothes, cleaning of weapons, and planning for the next stages of the journey. The Captains spent a lot of time writing reports, and Clark was always working on his map of the river that would incorporate all the observations made as they sailed along. But they also had other things to worry about.

Peace between the tribes was more difficult to achieve than Lewis and Clark realized. A message came that five Mandan warriors on a hunting party had been surprised by a group of Sioux. Whether the Sioux were on a war party or not was not explained, but one Mandan was killed, two were wounded, and nine horses were stolen. Clark wanted immediate retaliation. He gathered twenty-three men of the Corps and went to the Mandan village to help. The Mandans, not expecting such immediate powerful support, were surprised and thought the men of the Corps were coming to attack them. Clark explained that he wanted to help and "chastise the enemies of my dutiful children." He told them to send a runner to other villages and raise a bigger party. The Mandan Chiefs were more realistic and aware of the problems of winter warfare. They said that the snow was deep and cold, that the Sioux had fled, and anyway, their horses could not travel under these conditions. They said that if Clark would collect another party in the spring, when the conditions for war were better, they would go with him.

The Mandan Chiefs were smarter than Clark. Down the centuries, warfare in winter has been a disaster. From Xenophon's war campaign in 401 B.C. to the Battle of the Bulge and the Korean War the results have often been the same. After the retreat from Moscow in 1812, Napoleon said that he had not been defeated by the Czar Alexander but by the Generals January and February. During the depths of the winter the temperature near the Fort Mandan dropped to –40°F (–40°C). Add to that a powerful wind driving snow like bullets, and a vision rises of an Indian war party riding horses with their heads hanging low, blankets stiff with snow and ice drawn around the shoulders of the warriors, their lances gripped in frozen fingers, their war feathers a crown of ice. They could not have fought under any circumstances.

Cold was the enemy that Lewis and Clark had to fear. If they had sustained several serious cold injuries that left them with fewer men for the trip west they probably would have continued, but with a weakened party. If their chief hunters had been injured they would have been short of food. If their carpenters had been injured perhaps they would have had difficulty in building Fort Clatsop on the coast. If either Lewis or Clark had lost a foot to frostbite they might have continued, but with a weaker command.

Cold injures in many ways. The two most obvious injuries are frostbite and hypothermia. Frostbite is a local freezing of body tissues; hypothermia is general cooling of the whole body without freezing of tissue. It is possible to have frostbite without hypothermia and hypothermia without frostbite, but both are time and temperature related. The longer the exposure and the colder the temperature, the greater the chance of injury.

Lewis and Clark's men were not prepared to fight in winter. Every time they went out hunting they were in danger of being frostbitten. They had no fur clothing, no winter boots, and had not had time to make the clothes they lacked. The men came from warmer parts of the country, and although they had dealt with snow and cold weather, nothing could have prepared them for the bitterness and lethal cold of a Midwest blizzard. Clark's reaction to the Sioux foray was an act of bravado that could have been disastrous for the Corps. Fortunately, the Mandan Chiefs knew that in winter you stayed in your warm lodge, except to hunt, and did not go to war if you could avoid it.

Hippocrates knew that frostbite causes blisters similar to those caused by a burn, but the first physician to write a detailed description of frostbite and its treatment was the Baron Larrey, Surgeon-General to the Grand Army of Napoleon. He walked or rode every frozen mile back from Moscow to Poland and, after he returned, wrote a classic text about what he had seen. Sitting by the campfires

---

Most massive epidemics of frostbite have occurred in wars. In the fifth century B.C. Xenophon led his ragged army of ten thousand men through what is now Armenia, but lost two-thirds of them to frostbite and hypothermia. In 1812 Napoleon thought he could conquer Russia in twenty-two days and crossed the Niemen River in June with an army of six hundred thousand men. He reached Moscow with less than half his army and began to retreat in October. In November the first snow struck. One of Napoleon's aides described the scene. "Russian winter in this new guise attacked them on all sides: it cut through their thin uniforms and worn shoes, their wet clothing froze on them, and this icy shroud molded their bodies and stiffened their limbs." In December only a few thousand men staggered back across the Niemen. Hitler later made the same tactical mistake in 1941 and lost more than two hundred fifty thousand men to frostbite.

---

and watching the men die, dressing the frozen feet of soldiers, and helping the men across frozen rivers, he came to have strong opinions about the nature of frostbite and how it should be treated. "For it is well known that the effect of caloric on an organized part, which is almost deprived of life, is marked by an acceleration of fermentation and putrefaction." As he sat by the campfires and saw frozen legs and feet swell up and burst he came to believe that heat applied to a part already deprived of blood supply would only cause gangrene. The answer was to apply cold. Larrey, who was the first surgeon to design an ambulance for use on the battlefield, was a very influential figure in medicine and surgery. His opinion that frostbite should be treated by rubbing the frozen part with snow became the gospel by which patients were treated for more than a hundred years.

In the mid-1930s, two Russian scientists, S. S. Girgolav and T. J. Ariev, came to the conclusion that rubbing with snow did more harm than good. They carried out a series of experiments that showed warming was better treatment than cooling frozen tissue, as it led to the quickest recovery and the least damage. Their results were published in Russian medical journals and received no attention in the West, but their knowledge and experience were used later by the Russian Army.

When the United States entered the Second World War in 1941, research soon started at Stanford University to find a cure for frostbite. Professors J. M. Crismon and F. A. Fuhrman of the Department of Physiology were responsible for the research and soon found that it was easy to induce frostbite in animals. They found, like their Russian colleagues, whose work they had read, that rapid warming in warm water is the most effective treatment for frozen limbs. Their definitive paper on rapid rewarming was published in 1947. Within a few years this became the treatment accepted by NATO. Acceptance of the treatment by civilian doctors did not come until the 1960s when Dr. William Mills, an orthopedic surgeon in Anchorage, Alaska, published the first of many papers expounding his experience with rapid rewarming. In one form or another, this is now the accepted treatment for a frozen limb. Both principle and the practice are simple. The frozen part is soaked in water with a temperature between 100–105°F (39–45°C) and kept there for 30–40 minutes while color returns. If color and warmth return to the whole limb the result will be good. Parts of the limb that remain cold and white will probably become gangrenous.

Frostbite can be anything from a superficial nip that recovers without difficulty, to a massive freezing injury of a lower leg or whole hand, with subsequent loss of all the tissue that has been frozen. At first sight the frozen part is a pallid gray-white in color with no feeling. Blisters appear within a few hours on all but the most superficially frozen parts, usually on the fingers and toes. Blisters filled with bloody fluid are a bad sign and indicate significant damage and probable future loss of skin, at least, or the whole digit.

The management of severe frostbite is prolonged and difficult. Two to three weeks after the injury the skin becomes black and hard and the affected area begins to shrivel. If left alone, the part becomes gangrenous and—given time—separates spontaneously from the rest of the hand or foot. Immediately after the injury a doctor may find it difficult to tell what can be saved and what is going to be lost. The adage is "Frostbitten in January—amputate in July." Caution and conservative surgery are necessary to save as much tissue as possible. Even after the gangrenous parts have been removed there may be months of corrective surgery and rehabilitation. And the area remains sensitive to cold for the rest of the person's life, becoming painful and tingling whenever exposed to low temperatures.

During the course of the winter the men of the Corps had their fair share of exposure to cold and were at a continual risk for frostbite. They had to hunt, sometimes for days on end in bitter weather, and they often complained about their feet. Their first frostbite incident came in December 1804 when several men of a hunting group were badly frostbitten. The temperature was –44°F (–41°C).

The worst frostbite, however, occurred to the Indians. On January 10, 1805, the weather was extremely cold and the thermometer read –40°F. One of the men of the Corps had been out all night and returned uninjured, but the Indians borrowed a sled to look for a man and a boy who had not returned from the hunt. They expected to find both dead but, instead, brought in the boy with severely frostbitten feet and the man without any injury whatsoever.

> About 10 o'clock the boy about 13 years of age came to the fort with his feet frosed and had layen out all last night without fire with only a buffalo robe to cover him, the dress which he wore was a pair of antelope legins, which is verry thin and moccasins— we had his feet put in cold water and they are coming too—Soon after the arrival of the boy, a man came in who had also stayed out without fire, verry thinly clothed, this man was not the least injured—customs & the habits of thos people has ancered to bare more Cold than I thought it possible for a man to indure.

The boy's treatment was almost as good as could be given. His feet were put in cold water (which was warmer than the frozen feet, but was not as warm as would be used now) and some recovery began. Seventeen days later there was a brief note in Clark's journal. "Sawed off the boys toes." Lewis had already taken off the toes of one foot some days earlier. This operation was not as brutal and painful as might be thought. The tissues were already dead and without feeling and would have separated spontaneously if left alone.

Four days later some more toes were removed. The sequence of events suggests that Lewis understood when the toes were ready to be removed and did not remove any tissue that was still living. Six weeks after the boy was frostbitten his father came to the camp to take him home. Lewis recorded, "The father of the Boy whose feet were frose near this place, and nearly cured by us took him home in a slay."

Ideas about the underlying effects of frostbite have undergone important changes in the past few years. For most of the past one hundred years experts believed that the damage of frostbite was caused by the ice crystals that form between the cells. The tissue has to cool to between 25°F (−3.9°C) and 23°F (−5.0°C) for ice to form because the freezing point of the electrolyte-filled fluid of the tissues is lower than that of water. Sometimes supercooling, the process whereby the fluid remains unfrozen to an even lower temperature, results in tissues cooling to 20°F (–6.7°C). As the temperature of the tissues falls, the blood flow in the capillaries slows and the red cells, platelets, and white cells clump and plug up the small vessels. Local circulation comes to a halt. Under circumstances of normal body temperature, shutting off the circulation quickly results in cell death. But, when the cells are cold they are protected, just as they would be if put in the refrigerator. The protection is not perfect and some damage is done to the delicate intracellular structures while the cells are cold.

It was not until 1987 that two researchers in Chicago, John P. Heggers and Martin C. Robson, experts in the treatment of burns, investigated the similarity between the blisters of burns and the blisters of frostbite. They found that both blisters contained chemical breakdown products of what is now called "reperfusion injury." As the frozen parts rewarm, oxygen-carrying blood begins to flow through the capillaries and seep into the tissues. The damaged cells, however, react to the oxygen by swelling. Oxygen-starved cells do not react favorably, as might be expected, to the return of oxygen. The white blood cells become activated and produce chemical agents that induce constriction of capillaries. The blood flow that restarted with warming stops because of new tiny blood clots blocking the capillaries. The swelling of cells increases the pressure in the tissues, further restricting blood flow. These deleterious changes can be reversed by common anti-inflammatory agents. Although reperfusion causes some damage, rapid warming is, overall, better than allowing a frozen limb to cool spontaneously.

There is no magic cure for frostbite, but fortunately, there are now medications that counteract some of the damage to cells. Warming in water is still the foundation of treatment, but giving ibuprofen early in treatment may reduce the chances of some damage. If there is sufficient damage during cooling there may be no way to resurrect those cells. There is a borderline between the cells that are irretrievably damaged and those that are not damaged. And the objective of treatment is to save as many cells as possible in that shadow zone.

Rewarming may not be possible out in the field. One of the most disastrous situations is for a foot to be frozen, thaw, and then freeze for a second time. In this case, severe damage is certain. A frozen foot removed from a boot will swell and become painful as it warms, and it will be impossible to put the boot back on. Keeping the boot on and walking out on a frozen foot may cause less damage than allowing the foot to warm and be in danger of freezing again. Modern advice is to keep the frozen part cold until it can be rewarmed under circumstances in which further freezing is unlikely.

The treatment that Lewis gave to the Indian boy by putting his foot in cold water was surprisingly modern, and the only thing he could have done better would have been to place it in water warm enough for a baby's bath, but not hotter. The boy was fortunate that the foot did not refreeze. If that had happened he would have lost the whole foot.

The other great danger of cold is the development of hypothermia, generalized cooling of the body. Hypothermia is the opposite of heatstroke. In heat illness the body becomes hotter because it cannot dissipate the heat quickly enough. In hypothermia the body becomes cold because it cannot make, or retain, enough heat to counter the forces of heat loss. Hypothermia is not a problem of winter alone. Many mountain rescue groups see as many hypothermic victims in the summer as they do in winter. The cause is usually a combination of wind, wetness, and cold. Heat loss occurs about 25 times as fast through water as through air. Wetness is the enemy of heat. The mountain hiker who sets out on a bright summer day dressed in a T-shirt and shorts and without extra clothing may be heading for trouble. At noon the bright blue sky becomes cloudy, and an hour later there is a cold wind and driving rain. The T-shirt becomes soaked in a few seconds. The wind cools the skin. The body temperature falls. Within half an hour the person starts to shiver violently, becomes confused, and wants to rest, to sleep. The hiker cannot work a jacket zipper and stumbles on the trail. Hypothermia is developing rapidly. Shivering is the body's first defense against hypothermia. The metabolic rate and heat production can be increased five-fold by energetic shivering. Under some circumstances the body can produce more rewarming heat by shivering than can be provided by warm blankets. The time-honored method of putting a cold victim in a sleeping bag with a warm rescuer may not always be the best treatment. The rescuer's warmth may stop the cold person's shivering and slow rewarming. If the victim is shivering strongly it may be better to remove the wet clothes, put the person in a dry sleeping bag, and allow him or her to shiver themselves warm.

The correct immediate management of hypothermia is to get the victim out of the cold, the wind, and the rain. Remove cold, wet clothes, and dress the victim in dry clothes. If the person is awake and capable of eating, give them warm food and drink, not so much for the heat as for the renewed energy. A person who is severely hypothermic may be indistinguishable from someone who is dead. Their body is rigid, cold, motionless, and does not react to sensory stimulation. Perhaps the Indians who were left for dead by their companions were in that state. Becoming hypothermic on the plains near the Mandan village in 1805 would have been a catastrophe, and many braves and hunters must have perished in the winter blizzards. Lewis was astonished at the endurance of the Indians and their ability to withstand cold. The body can become physiologically acclimatized to heat, but there is no evidence that true acclimatization to cold can occur. Wearing few clothes from the time they were born, they became used to the cold and discomfort. They did, however, know that branches beneath them insulated them from the cold, and they slept with their feet toward the campfire, making sure that their feet did not become frostbitten.

Horses were also at risk for cold injuries. Winter was one of the hazards of a horse-based economy and culture. In the summer the horses had plenty of feed in the grass around the camps. In the winter there was no grass, feed was scarce, and the thin, poorly fed horses had a high mortality rate. Finding enough food to feed the horses was a serious problem. Most of the nomadic tribes that relied on horses kept eight to twelve horses per person. A tribal group of even a hundred people, therefore, kept hundreds of horses that had to be fed. The Mandans, being agriculturists, kept fewer horses and fed them the bark of cottonwood trees. This habit restricted the places where they could build their villages. Without logs for their houses, and without bark to feed their horses, they could not survive the winter.

Fort Mandan provided a warm base from which the Corps of Discovery could sortie to hunt and trade with the Indians. Hunting for food was a never-ending, difficult task. In February 1805, Clark recorded that their supplies of food were nearly exhausted. He set out with sixteen men, three packhorses, and two sleds (pulled by the men) and went to hunting grounds 60 miles away. The effort was worth the exertion. They killed forty deer, three bulls, and nineteen elk, but the animals were so thin that many of them were not used for food. No buffalo had appeared for some weeks, and the Indians were also wanting for food. The Chief, Black Cat, told Lewis he had not had any meat to eat for many days.

Hunting was seldom safe. Apart from the weather and the possibility of being stranded in a storm, marauding gangs of Sioux were a constant danger. Early in February Clark set out on another extended hunting trip. He proceeded down the frozen river for 22 miles and camped. The next day he fell through the ice and got his feet and legs wet, a dangerous accident, and one that could have led to serious frostbite. Clark and his party killed some deer and a skinny buffalo that were unfit for eating. He wrote that "walking on the uneven ice has blistered the bottom of my feet and walking is painful to me." A more likely explanation for the blisters is that, having gotten his feet wet, and not stopping to get into dry footwear, the soles of his feet were frostbitten. His feet had been mildly frostbitten a year before at Camp Dubois, and this previous exposure would not only have added to the likelihood of frostbite again, but would have sensitized his feet to the cold, making walking painful. The men wore moccasins, perhaps with double-thick soles for protection—we do not know. The insulation must have been poor unless they had made themselves larger boots and stuffed them with an inner lining of grass. The Indians were described as walking on thin moccasins, scanty protection against the cold, and the soldiers were probably not much better protected.

Every man in Clark's hunting party was engaged either in hunting or bringing the meat to the fort, now 44 miles away. Some of the meat was eaten by the wolves, ravens, and magpies that must have quickly become aware of the slaughter and taken the chance for an unexpected feast. The meat that was left at the hunting site was put in a pen for security. The party saw, and killed, more buffalo and grouse, and returned to the fort after ten days of travel. The day after returning four men were sent with shod horses (unshod horses could not travel on the ice and snow) and two sleds to get the meat that had been stored. They were rushed by a party of 106 Sioux who stole two of their three horses and much of the meat. They were allowed to keep one of the horses because a Sioux interceded on their behalf, probably being afraid of the revenge that might fall upon them. Lewis went out the next day with a party of soldiers and four Mandans, hoping to catch the Sioux. They had fled. The Indian guides surmised that the Sioux had been following the hunting party but had been afraid to attack. Half of the meat so laboriously shot and collected had been burned, but the Sioux failed to find one of the pens, and Lewis was able to return with 2,400 pounds of meat, having killed another thirty-six deer and fourteen elk.

On February 11, 1805, Sacagawea went into labor. This was her first child, and the labor was prolonged and difficult. René Jessaume, one of the interpreters, said that he had heard that giving a woman crushed-up rattle from a rattlesnake accelerated labor. Lewis had a rattle and ground up some of it and gave it to Sacagawea with some water. A fine baby boy was born within ten minutes. Lewis wrote in his journal, "Whether the medicine was truly the cause or not I shall not undertake to determine . . . perhaps this remedy may be worthy of future experiments, but I must confess that I want faith as to its efficacy." The substance of the rattle is similar to human fingernails, and many a mother must have chewed her nails during a long labor without any benefit. Lewis was right to be skeptical.

The birth of a child was the most notable medical event among their own people that Lewis and Clark had to deal with during the winter of 1804–1805. But there were plenty of lesser problems. The usual number of men reported "sick" and recovered without treatment. One man was "taken violently bad with the Plurisee, Bleed & apply those remedies common to that disorder." The remedies probably included Peruvian bark for the fever and laudanum for the pain. The man may also have been put in a sweat house.

At this time, Mr. Hugh Heney, an English trader with the North West Company, gave Lewis a plant—later identified as *Echinacea augustifolia*—that he said was magical in the treatment of bites from mad dogs and snakes. During the past few years both *Echinacea augustifolia* and *Echinacea purpurea* (purple coneflower) have become popular dietary supplements to cure and prevent the common cold. So far, there have been no reports of them being effective against snake- and mad-dog bites, although both plants have been shown to have properties that boost the immune system. Lewis later sent the plant to President Jefferson, but he never had occasion to use it himself.

In addition to these events many of the Indians came to the fort to receive medical treatment. Their gratitude was exemplified by the woman who brought her child with an abscess, carrying on her back, for payment, as much corn as she could lift. This exchange of medical treatment for food and other essentials continued throughout the voyage. Lewis, in his report to the President wrote, "The nations high up on the Missouri are Generly helthy but few of them have remidies for Disease, they make great use of the Coal bath & swets . . . the Goitre is common, womin perticularly." He made no mention of the high incidence of venereal disease among them and did not express any qualms about providing medical care to the Indians, as he did later in the voyage.

Later, as the days lengthened and the ducks and geese began to fly north in straggling chains, the men were set to chop out the barge and pirogues from the ice of the river and haul them up onto the bank—a task that required all of the energy they could muster. If they had waited until the spring breakup the boats would have been smashed between tumbling blocks of melting ice. The task took days. Finally the boats were free. The men placed log rollers beneath them, and hauling and straining on ropes made of elk skin, they pulled the boats up on the shore, out of the reach of the ice.

During the last few weeks of the stay in the fort both Lewis and Clark spent a lot of time writing. Lewis wrote a long report on the river and the state of the Indians, trying to answer many of the questions that had been posed to him by the President and Dr. Benjamin Rush. He commented on the animals and waterfowl, the different Indian tribes, their trade, their burial customs, what they were fond of—tobacco, guns, powder and ball, horses, knives, and spirits—their modes of punishment, how they buried their dead, and the contacts with British and French traders. He thought the traders were determined to put the worst possible light on the actions of the Americans, accusing them of giving the Indians a very unfavorable opinion of them.

Both Lewis and Clark sent Jefferson detailed reports about the Missouri River. Clark drew a map of the western half of the United States, making use of all the observations taken during the previous summer. The map of the Missouri as far as the Mandan villages was extremely accurate. Beyond that, much was conjecture, based on conversations with many Indians who liked to make three-dimensional maps in the sand, building the rivers, valleys, and mountains. Much of the information given was also very accurate, as many of the Indians had traveled across the plains as far as the Rocky Mountains, which the Hidatsas had penetrated on their raids.

Native people who do not rely on maps for finding their way often have photographic memories for the terrain they travel. Robert Marshall, an explorer of the Brooks Range in Alaska who lived in the small village of Wiseman for a year in the 1930s, recalled how an Eskimo girl was able to draw him a map of 40 miles of a river; a map so accurate she could describe exactly where individual trees were to be found. When Marshall traveled the river he found her description to be without fault. The problem Clark had to face was that there were no Indians who had gone all the way to the Pacific, and the descriptions on which he relied had to pass through two or three interpreters.

Lewis wrote nothing in his journal for several weeks before they left the fort; he was busy writing the other reports. Clark, as always, managed to write something, although his final entries were almost telegraphic in their brevity. "April 5th 1805 Thursday: we have our 2 perogues & six canoes loaded with our stores and provision, principally provisions. The wind verry high from the NW. A number of Mandans visit us today." On the same date Sergeant Ordway wrote that it was a clear, pleasant day and it was spent sorting and loading. The following day, one day before they left, there was obviously some excitement that a large band of Arikaras had appeared on the other side of the river. Ordway noted that the officers wanted to wait and find out what was happening. Fortunately, all was well and the Arikaras had arrived because some of them wanted to go to St. Louis.

After the winter at Fort Mandan, Lewis and Clark organized the final members of the expedition. The main party, to advance up the river and to the West Coast, consisted of the two Captains; three Sergeants; two interpreters; twenty-two Privates; Clark's slave, York; Charbonneau's wife, Sacagawea and her infant son, Baptiste; and one big, friendly dog, Seaman. In accordance with the plan that had been prepared for a long time, Corporal Warfington was to lead a group of six Privates, four engagés, and an Arikara Indian back downriver in the keelboat and a small canoe. They took with them letters, reports, mineral and biological specimens, and six live animals. Four magpies, a prairie dog, and a short-tailed grouse were packed into crates to be sent to Jefferson, who liked to receive live gifts. Two years later Zebulon Pike sent a pair of grizzly bear cubs that proved to be too rambunctious for the White House. They were passed on to a zoo in Philadelphia from which one of them escaped. By that time it weighed 300 pounds and scared the life out of the people in the Philosophical Hall where it sought refuge. It had to be shot. Only one magpie survived the journey to Washington and proved to be much less of a problem than a grizzly bear cub.

The morning of April 7, 1805, the day of departure, was a very busy time. The Captains were making last-minute contact with the

Indians and supervising the loading of the pirogues and canoes. The men must have been wondering if they had brought everything they would need. Could they pack in one last detail? There would be no turning back and no resupply. Lewis later wrote in his journal: "Having on this day at 4pm completed every arrangement necessary for our departure, we dismissed the barge and crew with orders to return without loss of time to St Louis. . . . we have therefore every hope that the barge with our dispatches will arrive safe at St Louis." The words that Lewis wrote about his own departure must stand as some of the finest ever written in the literature of exploration.

> Our vessels consisted of six small canoes, and two large pirogues. This little fleet altho' not quite so respectable as those of Columbus or Captain Cook, were still viewed by us with as much pleasure as those deservedly famed adventurers ever beheld theirs; and I dare say with as much anxiety for their safety and preservation. We were now about to penetrate a country at least two thousand miles in width, on which the foot of civilized man had never trodden; the good or evil it had in store for us was for experiment yet to determine, and these little vessels contained every article by which we were to expect to subsist or defend ourselves.

Lewis had already written a letter to the President and another to his mother. He was in a writing mood, and the importance of the moment, his dreams and hopes, and his confidence in the outcome all came bubbling to the surface. "At this moment, every individual of the party are in good health and excellent sperits; zealously attached to the purpose, and anxious to proceed; not a whisper of discontent of murmur to be heard among them; but all in unison, act with the most perfect harmoney. With such men I have everything to hope, but little to fear."

The two parties made their last farewells, waved to each other, and pushed off in opposite directions. One group back to the comforts of home. The other to an unknown fate in an unknown land.

SIX

All Go Cheerfully On:
April–November 1805

66 "I could but esteem this moment of our departure as among the most happy of my life." So wrote Lewis on April 7, 1805, in a long entry in his journal after they had embarked on the most adventurous endeavor of their voyage. Before them stretched 2,000 miles of unknown territory. The Indians at Fort Mandan had filled in many of the gaps in their knowledge, but the route was still fraught with incalculable difficulties and dangers. The men had no idea of the magnitude of the mountains, their height and breadth and ruggedness. They did not know if the Shoshone (Snake) Indians would be friendly and if they would be able to get horses from them. Without horses their task would have been impossibly difficult. They knew nothing of the distance between the rivers that flowed east and west, but they hoped it would be a simple portage between one river and another. They did not even know if the river to the ocean would be navigable.

Some facts were known. They knew that the Missouri had several tributaries, such as the Yellowstone River, and they learned about high waterfalls that would obstruct their progress. They had been told that the Missouri divided into several branches, but they did not know which branch would be the most advantageous route into the mountains. They had heard of various Indian tribes they might encounter but did not know if they would be friendly or warlike. In spite of all this uncertainty, Lewis could regard this as one of the happiest days of his life. They were off again on what he called the "darling project of mine for the last ten years."

Spring was just around the corner. Birds were migrating, buds and roots were sprouting, and those harbingers of summer, the mosquitoes, were already a pest, but not as bad as they would be later on. Large flocks of Canada and snow geese were feeding on the river bottom, and they found—to their surprise—that some of the geese nested high in the cottonwood trees. The sharp-tailed grouse were drumming and mating. In places the river was filled with the carcasses of buffalo that had fallen through the melting ice and drowned. In the sand around the carcasses they saw tracks of enormous "white" bears, as the grizzly was called. Immense herds of buffalo, elk, deer, and antelope spread over the plains. The river-banks were full of beaver, and they encountered three French trappers hunting for furs: the forerunners of those who would come after and deplete the river of all its beaver.

The Captains took turns walking along the shore, sometimes exploring many miles from the river. They tasted the water of small streams and found it to be brackish and full of minerals, "like Glauber salts." Clark came across the disused camp of an Assiniboine group. He assumed that it had been an Assiniboine camp because the remains of rum kegs were scattered around the huts. The Assiniboines were very fond of rum supplied to them by the British, and according to Lewis, they did not think that getting drunk was a cause for shame. If they had enough rum the whole tribe would become intoxicated, including the women and children. In return for the rum the Assiniboines sold wolf and fox furs to the traders.

Travel on the river was not any easier than it had been before. The white pirogue, believed to be the most stable of all the craft, was loaded with the most precious instruments and cargo. Just a few days out it was proceeding "at a pretty good gate" under a small square sail and a spritsail. A sudden squall of wind nearly tipped it over, and Charbonneau, who was at the helm, panicked and allowed it to get beam on to the wind. Lewis yelled at the reliable Drewyer to take over the helm and drop the sail. This was done, control was regained, and all was saved. Lewis developed a poor opinion of Charbonneau as a helmsman, and called him "the most timid waterman in the world."

A month later Charbonneau was involved in a similar accident on the river, losing control of the pirogue while both Lewis and Clark were on shore and unable to help. Once again the pirogue was turned beam on to the wind, and, instead of permitting it to be turned around and sail before the wind, Charbonneau luffed it into the wind. The boat was nearly turned "topsaturva," and Charbonneau allowed the pirogue to lie on its side, nearly sinking. Lewis was on the point of taking off his jacket and trying to swim the 300 yards to the boat to set things right. Fortunately, he thought better of his folly, which might have cost him his life, and Cruzatte took control, threatening to shoot Charbonneau if he did not take hold of the rudder. All the while Charbonneau, who could not swim, was crying to his God for mercy. Clark wrote, "We owe the preservation of the pirogue to the resolution and fortitude of Cruzatte." Lewis gave equal praise to Sacagawea: "The Indian woman, to whom I ascribe equal fortitude and resolution with any person onboard at the time of the accident, caught and preserved most of the light articles which were washed overboard."

That evening, Lewis thought the thrills of the day warranted some extra cheer. "After having all matters arranged for the evening as well as the nature of the circumstances would permit, we thought it a proper occasion to console ourselves and cheer the sperits of our men and accordingly took a drink of grog and gave each man a gill of sperits."

Maintaining morale was important and not always easy. Sometimes the men were up to their armpits in the water; at others, they were slipping and sliding along muddy banks, or trying to find a foothold with bare feet on a rocky shore or across a grass slope filled with prickly pear cactus. "Their labour is incredibly painfull and great, yet those faithfull fellows bear it without a murmur."

There had to be times of relief. Cruzatte played his fiddle. The Captains gave out a dram of whiskey, and the men danced and sang long into the night, forgetful of their sore and bleeding feet. If only

Lewis or Clark had written down the hilarious stories that must have been told, the ribald jokes, the old, favorite songs. There is a companionship between people all experiencing the same hard times and grim circumstances that transcend all other friendships. Lewis repeatedly referred to Clark in glowing terms as his "worthy" friend. The journals give no hint of angry words, or even angry thoughts between the two. There were things that Lewis liked that Clark did not, such as dog meat, but their differences of opinion were amazingly mild and were never differences involving command. The unity and stability of the expedition depended not only on friendship and trust, but also the recognition of who was in command.

There was never any doubt that Lewis was the commander. Later, on the way home, the expedition split into parties with Lewis in charge of one group, Clark in charge of another, and Sergeant Ordway in charge of a third. But each man knew his place and his responsibilities. Each man knew that the other would do his job for the greater good of the expedition. The crew knew that the Captains had their welfare at heart. Both Lewis and Clark were physicians to the men, although the Indians seemed to prefer Clark as their doctor. He had a better tent-side manner. Although Clark had been promised a Captain's rank he was only given a Lieutenant's badge. Lewis never accepted this and called him Captain. As far as the crew was concerned they were both Captains, of equal rank but with different responsibilities. If they had not been equal partners the hierarchy of the group would have been different. As it was, the arrangement worked to perfection.

Both Captains proved themselves under many circumstances. Lewis calmed one of the soldiers who had slipped over the edge of a cliff and quietly instructed him to take out his knife with his spare hand—the other hand was hanging on for dear life—and make a foothold in the slippery surface. Both survived. Clark was the persuasive leader when the expedition was in the Rockies, approaching the first Indian group they had seen for months. Once, while Lewis was ahead negotiating with the Indians, Clark persuaded the men to make the last efforts to drag the canoes through an increasingly cold, narrow, rocky stream because relief, rest, and horses to carry the loads were just ahead. He was walking in extreme pain with a large abscess on his ankle when he might have demanded time to rest. The men saw these things and knew that they could do nothing less themselves. The leadership, by example, was followed willingly.

In spite of the rugged conditions and unknown prospects, Lewis and Clark only twice expressed doubt. Lewis, on his thirty-first birthday on August 18, 1805, confided to his journal that he doubted what he had achieved and his commitment to the human race and vowed to do better. When they had reached the coast and were perched on the rocks under the most miserable, rainy, cold circumstances, Clark let his fortitude slip for a moment. "O! how disagreeable is our situation dureing this dreadfull weather. We are all wet bedding and stores, having nothing to keep ourselves or stores dry, our Lodge nearly worn out and the pieces of sales & tents so full of holes & rotten that they will not keep anything dry. . ." An understandable complaint. Only an idiot or a supreme masochist would not have complained and pretended that everything was fine. However, the truth was that, at that moment, there was no alternative.

As the group proceeded farther and farther up the Missouri, new problems arose. Many of the men broke out in the boils that had plagued them in the first part of the trip to the Fort Mandan. It has been suggested that the men were suffering from malnutrition and were susceptible to infections. Until they reached the Great Falls, which were still several months away, food was in abundance, including fresh meat and fruits. But they were in water every day, and their skin, although toughened, must have become waterlogged and subject to multiple cuts and abrasions. Their clothes were rough buckskin and filthy—ready sources of infection. One man got an abscess alongside his fingernail that made work on the boats very painful.

Sore eyes also troubled many of the men. Not long after leaving Fort Mandan sand and dust were blowing across the river and infiltrating everything, including their eyes. They had neither sunglasses nor goggles to protect their eyes. Their eyes must have been red, scratchy, and bleary; a constant source of irritation. Clark had "eye water" in the medical kit, but little is said about giving it to the men, although it was later distributed liberally to the Nez Percé Indians.

In addition, two animals posed greater problems than in the first stage of the journey: rattlesnakes and bears. Almost as soon as they started into new country, rattlesnakes became common, and, when walking in the grass, the men had to keep their eyes and ears open. In one area near the Great Falls, Clark described the rattlesnakes as innumerable and wrote that everyone had to be very careful. Fortunately, no one was bitten, although there were many close encounters, some of them scary. Joseph Whitehouse was struck on the leg, but as he was wearing thick leather leggings the fangs did not penetrate and he was not envenomated. The snake was large, 4 feet 10 inches long, and more than 5 inches in circumference. The longest prairie rattler caught in modern times was 57 inches long. The snake that struck Whitehouse was record-size. During the extraordinary portage around the Great Falls, when the men were struggling to haul homemade wagons with heavy loads across rough country, one of them reached out to grab a branch for better purchase and found that he had grasped a rattlesnake. It did not strike. Lewis awoke one morning to find a very large rattlesnake coiled on a branch about 10 feet from him. The snake did not attack, and Lewis killed and measured it, as he did with so many animals. His curiosity never flagged.

Rattlesnakes are pit vipers, a family with a small heat-sensing pit near the tip of the nose. This organ, which is anatomically similar to the middle ear, except that it senses heat rather than sound, enables the snake to recognize when a warm-blooded animal is within about 2 feet. This information enables the snake to strike with accuracy and to localize its victims in the dark. If a rattlesnake is experimentally irritated with two balloons, one filled with cold water and the other filled with water at body temperature, it will always strike at the warm balloon. The flicking tongue is the organ by which the snake tracks its victims with a combination of taste and smell, until the heat-sensing pit indicates when the prey is close enough to strike. When the snake strikes, its mouth opens wide so that the fangs, normally tucked under the upper jaw, swing into the attack position. The venom is stored in sacs alongside the upper jaw and is squeezed into the victim through fangs that function like hypodermic needles. Sometimes the snake misses, or the fangs do not enter the victim, or, because the snake has just emptied its poison sacs, the bite is "dry." A quarter of all bites fail to inject venom.

Rattlesnakes are still common in the areas through which the expedition passed and are much more common than the average citizen might believe. Snakes like to lie quietly and, unless disturbed, may not give any sign of their presence. As a rattlesnake can only strike over a distance equal to about half its body length, it is possible to walk near a snake without being in serious danger of being bitten. This relatively short striking distance is the reason that most bites occur on the legs below the knee, or on the hands of people reckless enough to reach blindly into holes. There are about eight thousand snakebites every year in the United States, but only about ten deaths. In contrast, there are about twenty thousand deaths every year from cobra bites in India, and about sixty thousand snakebite deaths per year worldwide.

Part of the low rattlesnake-bite mortality is due to modern treatment with antivenin, but part is due to the nature of rattlesnake venom compared with the venom of the Indian cobra or the Australian brown snake. Rattlesnake venom primarily causes local damage, and systemic damage, such as the cessation of respiration, a late effect in very severe bites. One investigator found that, in fatal rattlesnake bites, the average time between bite and death was six to eight hours, plenty of time, in most cases, to get the victim to treatment. Cobra venom acts much more quickly and stops respiration and cardiac action, sometimes within minutes, by acting on the nervous system. Even at the time of the Lewis and Clark expedition a tourniquet, incision, and suction were advocated as a way to extract the venom and effect a cure. Experts now advise against a tourniquet unless it is applied gently enough to stop only the flow of lymph, and does not stop arterial flow. If it is too tight and kept on too long, shutting off the circulation severely damages the limb.

Some experts say, half jokingly, that the best treatment for snakebites is to own a car and a set of car keys. Lewis never used any native cures for snakebites, but he did apply gunpowder to the bitten area, a common "cure" of the time.

Many useless, and sometimes dangerous, treatments have been advocated for snakebites, including shocking the area with electricity from the cigarette lighter in your car, or freezing the bite with immersion in ice water. If symptoms develop quickly with increasing swelling of the bitten limb, evidence of shock, and a fall in blood pressure or unconsciousness, antivenin in large volumes, given intravenously, is the only hope of saving life and limb.

Rattlesnakes, as opposed to some snakes in other parts of the world, are not aggressive. Most will try to escape rather than attack. The sibilant rattle is a warning to stay away and is not a sign of immediate attack. It is a noise that must have become familiar to the men of the Corps. The large snake that Lewis killed probably would have slithered away without doing any harm if it had been given the chance. But it would take a very patient, snake-savvy person to watch it quietly depart, and few people would blame Lewis for killing it. Attitudes toward rattlesnakes, however, are changing slowly. The huge rattlesnake roundups are disappearing for the good ecological reason that if too many snakes are killed, the population of rodents will increase accordingly. But Lewis did not live in an era of ecological sensitivity. He followed natural instincts that were as old as the Garden of Eden.

The second animal that caused alarm was the grizzly bear. The Indians had warned the expedition about the "white" bear, impressing on the men how difficult they were to kill. The men saw huge grizzly footprints along the shore of the river, but, at first, did not have any close encounters. Several bears were spotted far away and they all fled. This caused Lewis to think that perhaps the Indians had been exaggerating and that the bears were actually nervous and shy. Lewis thought that the men would have considerable sport hunting the bears and scoffed at the opinion the Indians had of the big creatures. After shooting the first grizzly on April 29, 1805, Lewis wrote that the Indians, armed with bows and arrows and imperfect "fusees" might fear these bears, but "in the hands of a skilful rifleman they are by no means as formidable or dangerous as they have been represented." It did not take long for him to change his mind.

Six days later Drewyer shot a "very large and terrible-looking" bear that took ten rifle balls to kill it. In another six days, William Bratton, who had been excused of duties on the boat because of a sore hand, came running back to the river. He had shot at a bear that chased him for more than half a mile despite bleeding from its lungs. Lewis took seven men to hunt for the animal and eventually found it, still alive, in a trough it had dug for itself. They dispatched it with a shot through the head. Two days later another bear was wounded but not pursued.

May 11, 1805, the day when Charbonneau nearly lost the pirogue for a second time, was wild and dangerous. That same evening, six of the men, all good hunters, who had seen a large grizzly lying 300 hundred yards away from the river, ventured forth to kill it. They managed to get within 40 yards of the bear before four of them fired at it simultaneously, while two held their fire in reserve. The bear came at them, roaring, and the two with loaded guns in reserve, fired. One bullet broke the bear's shoulder, a wound that only stopped it for a moment. The bear chased the men to the river where two of them retreated to a canoe, while the others hid in the bushes, reloading their guns. The bear was struck again, several times, but, suddenly realizing this new assault was coming from the bushes, turned and chased the two men into the river. The bear plunged into the river after one of the men and nearly caught him. The last hunter, who had reloaded, shot the bear through the head and killed it. Eight balls had passed through the bear, which was old and thin and unsuitable for eating. The men no longer thought that the white bears were shy and retiring.

"I must confess I do not like the gentleman and had rather fight two Indians than one bear; there is no other chance to conquer them by a single shot but by shooting them through the brains." Lewis realized how difficult this is to do because of the thickness of the muscles filling the temples and a ridge of thick bone that runs down the center of the skull. Many a hunter since has found the same difficulty.

Grizzly bears had not been a threat in the first stage of the journey, and it was only after leaving Fort Mandan that the first "white bear" was seen. The journals record thirty-seven close meetings with grizzlies within four months, a number that even experienced hunters in Alaska would not expect to have in a lifetime in the wilderness. Through good luck and the natural behavior of bears, no one was hurt or killed. Shooting and wounding an animal as huge, short-tempered, and powerful as a grizzly bear is not the way to scare it away. Its rage will be immediate and ferocious.

From 1900 to 1979 there were nineteen deaths from grizzly bear attacks in the lower United States and another twenty-two in Alaska. Since then there have been fewer than four deaths per year in the entire Unites States, including Alaska. In Yellowstone National Park there is about one injury for every million and a half visitors. Considering the number of hikers, hunters, and wilderness

---

While traveling in Alaska, I was standing with friends by a stream in the Brooks Range when we saw a grizzly, of moderate size, come wandering down the valley, minding its own business and flipping over rocks, looking for ground squirrels. Suddenly, 50 yards away, it became aware of our smell and stood on its hind legs to get a better look at us. To our eyes it immediately changed from a small bear to one that looked 30 feet tall. To our relief it dropped to all fours and charged away across the river—golden evening spray flying around it. The bear kept on running up the boulder-covered hill as though the slope was a flat sidewalk, leaving behind an indelible impression of power and speed. The adrenaline rush on seeing a grizzly at close quarters is never forgotten.

wanderers who have trekked through the national parks and the territories of the bears in the same period, the number of attacks and deaths has been extraordinarily small. Bear attacks are "provoked" or "unprovoked." Most of the attacks against the men of the expedition were provoked maximally. Lewis and Clark thought the bears were immensely dangerous, so dangerous that Lewis forbade the men to venture alone into the brush where bears were common. Wandering quietly through thick bushes in grizzly country is dangerous. If bears are warned by approaching people, like the rattlesnakes, they will usually retreat.

There are places in Alaska along the Brooks and McNeil rivers where the bears have become so habituated to humans that they will walk calmly, within a few yards of people, fully aware of them, and confident that these strange-smelling bipeds will do them no harm. In other areas where the bears have been hunted their behavior is different. They are cautious, as shy as Lewis thought, but occasionally aggressive. Lewis experienced this when he was chased into the river and the bear came to the shore, looked at Lewis, and turned away. Lewis concluded that the bear did not want to do battle with him. Lewis was right, but for the wrong reasons. Lewis thought the bear was afraid. In fact, the bear probably thought he had chased away a bothersome pest and could go about the much more interesting business of eating a dead buffalo.

Many charges by grizzlies are bluffs. The bear hurls itself at the intruder and then, at the last minute, turns away to the side. Many grizzlies, shot by hunters while charging, received a fatal shot in the side of the chest. If the bear had still been coming directly at the hunter at the moment of death, the wound would have been found in the front of the chest or head. A side shot in the chest means that the bear had already turned away when it was shot.

Most of the bears that the men of the expedition encountered had never seen or smelled a human before. The sights and smells of humans were a new experience for them. If the bears thought the men were threatening their territory or their food they might charge, and, if the bear had been a mother with cubs—and none of the attacks described in the journals involved a mother with cubs—a charge would have been very likely. Grizzlies don't like to be surprised, and coming upon a bear in thick brush is a likely scenario for an attack. On at least one occasion the men went into thick willows, looking for a bear they had seen or wounded. Considering the relatively small power of their rifles and the time it took to reload, this was extremely dangerous, and they were lucky not to be attacked and killed.

The front claws of a grizzly are massive, powerful digging instruments. A swipe across the face from a bear removes half the tissues, bone, and skin. If a bear reaches for someone trying to escape by climbing a tree, there is not much meat left on the person's back. Grizzlies do not climb trees, as their cousins the black bears do, but standing on its hind legs a large bear can reach 10 feet up into a tree. Anyone trying to escape the attack of a grizzly by climbing a tree has to get high enough to keep their legs out of reach. One man was treed and sat for a long time with a snorting, unhappy bear prowling around the foot of his refuge. He probably knew that grizzlies do not climb trees, but he must have spent an uneasy time expecting an unwelcome visitor beside him at any moment.

On May 26, 1805, Lewis saw the Rocky Mountains for the first time. He had mixed feelings: "When I viewed these mountains I felt a secret pleasure . . . but when I reflected on the difficulties which this snowey barrier would probably throw in my way to the Pacific, and the sufferings of myself and party in them, it in some measure counter ballanced the joy I felt in the first moments in which I gazed on them."

The land they were passing through was well known to the roving, nomadic Indians, but even Sacagawea, who had been brought from the Rockies to the Missouri valley, did not know exactly where they were. She had made the journey by land, along a different route. The Corps would have to travel many miles before they reached land that was familiar to her. What a different journey this was for Sacagawea. Instead of being hounded along, a slave and prisoner, she was now part of an expedition, protected by forty armed men and was heading to her home territory. We learn almost nothing about her emotions from the journals. Lewis thought that all she needed were a few trinkets and she would be happy under any circumstances, good or bad. Yet, when she finally met with her family, the tears flowed and she became as emotional as Lewis himself might have become in the same situation. She could not speak English, although it is hard to believe she did not pick up some of the language as the voyage progressed. If language was a barrier, there was no one to whom she could express her thoughts and emotions except through interpreters. She had no sister with her, and there were no other wives. She was in a world of rough, tough men with a small baby to look after. Feeding the baby was not a problem as Baptiste had still not been weaned, even by the end of the trip, a year later. Benjamin Rush had wanted to know how long Indian mothers breast-fed their babies, and, in Sacagawea's case, the answer was at least eighteen months. This habit protected the babies. The adult's food was dirty and poorly cooked, and the incidence of diarrhea in small Indian children after they were weaned must have been high, as it is today in third-world countries. Breast-feeding for a long time was the cleanest, healthiest way to nourish the children.

From the time they left the Mandans until they met the Shoshones in the Rockies, the expedition did not meet any Indians for several weeks. Signs of Indian hunting parties were everywhere, but the natives had passed on to other hunting grounds, some of them recently. Abandoned huts and fireplaces indicated that the Indians were not far away. The Corps were not passing through an empty land, just one in which the inhabitants were moving, cautious and concealed. The absence of encounters relieved the Corps of many worries. Because much of the country was treeless and wide open they would have been able to see parties of Indians, but they could have missed a careful Indian scout watching them from a distance. Word of the expedition was certain to have passed between the Indians, and rumors must have been flying in the Indian camps about the large group of white men traveling on the river. Did the Indians leave them alone because they did not want to get into a fight? Or, were they too busy hunting to be bothered with a group they did not see as an immediate threat? The Indians left no records of their thoughts, but Lewis and Clark were glad not to meet an aggressive war party.

During this stretch of the trip, the general health of the men remained good, but problems were always arising. A month after leaving the Mandans Joseph Fields became very sick with dysentery and a high fever. Lewis gave Fields a dose of Glauber's salts "which operated very well, and in the evening he felt better." This incident was typical of many episodes of gastrointestinal illness. One man would become sick for a day and, usually in response to a laxative, get better. We would now call this "traveler's diarrhea," a brief, sometimes explosive attack of diarrhea that lasts for twenty-four to forty-eight hours and usually disappears without drastic treatment. The usual definition of traveler's diarrhea is more than three loose stools in a twenty-four-hour period. The diarrhea is often accompanied by nausea, vomiting, and cramping abdominal pain. Not the symptoms one would like to have while exploring a river on boats. On one occasion Charbonneau was sick, and Lewis allowed him to walk on shore, probably for the practical reason that it was not possible to stop the boat frequently to allow a crew member to retire into the bushes. If the diarrhea continues for several days the worst problem may be dehydration and loss of electrolytes in the watery stools. Replacement of fluids is an important part of treatment. In the extreme diarrheal diseases, such as cholera, the victims can die from dehydration, if not cured by drinking electrolyte replacement fluids. The World Health Organization has designed packets of sugar and electrolytes that can easily be mixed with sterile water and given to patients. This simple treatment has saved millions of lives in third-world countries where infantile and childhood diarrhea is a major cause of death.

The common form of traveler's diarrhea is most often caused by *Escherichia coli,* an organism universally resident in the bowel. There are many different strains of the bacterium, some of which have caused lethal outbreaks. Most of these episodes have arisen from improperly handled and cooked meat. We do not know what bacterial strains were prevalent among the men of the expedition or in the Indians with whom they mixed. Many of the intestinal complaints could have been due to viruses. The so-called enteroviruses are a very common cause of intestinal disease in modern times, accounting for ten to twelve million cases of diarrhea in the United States every year. If the stools become bloody and high fever continues for a few days, then the illness may be due to an invasive organism such as *shigella*. Later in the voyage, after struggling through the worst of the mountains, most of the men were afflicted with diarrhea. Although the men ascribed the problem to a change in diet, it is much more likely that they became infected with some organism from their own or the Indians' food. The conditions for an epidemic were perfect: a group of cold, wet, exhausted, poorly fed, stressed-out men, eager to eat anything put in front of them and eating a diet of roots and dried fish that was foreign to them.

During these months a series of accidents occurred, fortunately none of them serious, but some that potentially could have ended in disaster. Charbonneau seemed to have been born under an ill-fated star. He was involved in several accidents on the river. He was not a man of courage and calmness and reacted to a crisis with alarm and panic. Twice he nearly caused a serious accident with the boats. He was chased by a bear and fled, firing his gun into the air. He, Clark, and Sacagawea and Baptiste were nearly killed in a flash flood. They were walking down a ravine when an upstream rainstorm made the creek rise 15 feet in a few minutes. A surge of muddy water nearly swept them away. They scrambled up the steep bank and hung precariously until they could pull themselves to safety.

Sergeant Pryor dislocated his shoulder for the second time. When a shoulder dislocates the capsule around the joint is sometimes torn, making it easy for the bone to pop out of the joint on a future occasion. This is probably what happened with Pryor, and the second time, it was easy to reduce the dislocation.

When the expedition was near the Three Forks of the Missouri one of the canoes swung wildly in the river, tipping Whitehouse into the water. His foot caught on the bottom of the stream and the boat swung back over him. In his diary he wrote that his leg was nearly broken, and he was swept under the boat and nearly drowned. Poor unlucky Charbonneau also nearly drowned in another incident, but he was saved by Clark.

Nighttime carried its own dangers. One night a tree standing close to the tent in which Lewis, Clark, and others were sleeping caught fire and nearly fell across the tent. If the burning tree had not been seen, several people might have died. On another occasion, a buffalo wandered through camp, probably unconcerned at first, but then alarmed by Seaman, Lewis' dog, barking a warning. The dog chased the buffalo away from the sleepers.

Contrary to superstition, June 13, 1805, did not bring Lewis bad luck. It was a banner day: one he would remember for the rest of his life. Two days earlier he had set out with a small party, in advance of the main group, to explore the branch of the river that he and Clark thought was the main trunk of the Missouri. There had been a discussion among the group at the point where the river divided. The men thought the northern branch would lead them to the mountains. Lewis and Clark thought the southern branch was the one to follow. If Lewis was correct, he would find the waterfalls the Indians had described to him.

He shouldered his pack—a task he was not used to—and, after a breakfast of venison and fish, climbed the hills to flat prairie. As he and his men came over the rise a plain of 50 to 60 miles in extent opened in front of them, adorned with two buttes, each about 250 feet high. Fields was sent to the right, Drewyer and George Gibson to the left, and Silas Goodrich was told to stay a short distance behind. All were ordered to hunt for meat; not a difficult job as the plain was thick with buffalo. Lewis proceeded ahead by himself. He began to hear the sound of rushing water. Soon he saw spray, rising like steam above the flatland. The noise changed from a distant rumble to a roar, and, at noon, having walked about 15 miles since breakfast, he overlooked the Great Falls, a sight he called "this sublimely grand spectacle." The description he wrote in his journal is long and lyrical. He wrote of the rocks, the sparkling foam, the rolling bodies of beaten, foaming water. He ran out of words and nearly scrapped the whole description, yearning for the words of a poet and the pen of an artist to describe what he had seen.

Lewis made his camp under a tree and sent one of the men to tell Clark what he had found and to look for a suitable landing place downstream from the falls. That evening they dined like kings— buffalo hump, tongues and marrow, cutthroat trout broiled in meal, and enjoyed a good appetite. Only three days before Lewis had been sick and dining on a decoction of chokecherry to settle his stomach.

The next day four other falls came into view farther up the river. Another that was equal in beauty to the first he called "pleasingly beautiful." He was on a visual high. He climbed a small hill from which he could look downstream and upstream along the length of the Missouri. "I also observed the missoury stretching its meandering course to the south through this plain to a great distance filled to its even and grassey brim." A bald eagle was nesting on a small island above the uppermost fall, and vast flocks of geese bobbed on the smooth river above the falls. It was no wonder that Lewis wanted the words of a poet.

The day was not finished. Knowing that he had to camp and eat, Lewis shot a buffalo and stood watching attentively as blood poured from the dying animal's nostrils and mouth. He was so intrigued by this sight that he did not reload his gun and failed to notice a grizzly stalking him until it was only 20 feet away. There was nowhere to hide. The plain was flat and the nearest bush was 300 yards away. He looked around desperately and saw a distant tree and started to walk quickly toward it. Within seconds he was running for his life, the bear rapidly closing in on him. Realizing that the tree was beyond his reach, he made for the river, hoping that he could reach a depth where the bear would have to swim, but he could stand and defend himself. He plunged into the river and went 20 feet from the shore and turned to meet his pursuer. The bear "suddenly wheeled about as if frightened, declined the combat on such unequal grounds, and retreated with quite as great precipitation as he had just before pursued me." Lewis went back up on the bank and watched the bear flee at full speed across the plain. Later, Lewis pondered about the bear's behavior. He examined the ground where the bear had chased him and saw the marks of its talons as it ripped up the earth in pursuit. He found the situation "misterious and unaccountable." The bear, driven by a hunting instinct, chased him because he ran away. Then, when Lewis went in the river, the bear, having made a bluff charge and happy to be rid of the intruder, decided to leave the scene. Lewis learned an important lesson: he was never again going to be left with an unloaded gun. He walked all day and arrived back at camp to find his men anxious for his safety and wondering if he might have been killed. He was fatigued but ate a hearty supper and settled down for a good rest.

As soon as Lewis returned to the main camp he learned that Sacagawea was very ill with severe abdominal pain and had not responded to the treatment Clark had started. He immediately took her history, examined her, and was justifiably alarmed. Her pulse was rapid, weak, and irregular, and he was afraid she might die. For whatever reasons, she was in the early stages of shock. He referred to her, somewhat impersonally in the journals as "the Indian woman." His concern for her was genuine, not only as a person, but he knew that if she died the future of the expedition might be jeopardized. She was the essential link to the Shoshones who would be the suppliers of horses. Without horses it would be virtually impossible to cross the Rockies.

Lewis attributed Sacagwea's illness to obstructed menses "due to cold." It was remarkable that he asked Sacagawea about her menstrual history, because there was a language barrier between the two of them and because most men of that time would not have asked women about such an intimate detail. It is remarkable in another way because Clark had been concerned about how hot, not how cold, she was, lying in the bottom of the pirogue.

A physician can surmise from the journal entries that Sacagawea was suffering from peritonitis of the lower part of her abdomen. This could have been due to inflammation of the uterus or fallopian tubes and may have been a flare-up of a previous infection, although there was no evidence from the journals that she had been suffering from discomfort in the previous weeks. The language barrier and her innate stoicism may have prevented her from talking about her symptoms.

Once again, imagination has overcome logic in the minds of some historians who have construed the diagnosis as a venereal disease contracted when she was purportedly raped by the Hidatsas. Yet, there is no evidence that Charbonneau subsequently contracted a venereal disease from his wife.

She was bled and purged in an attempt to cure her, and there is little doubt that this must have weakened and dehydrated her, as well as upset the balance of electrolytes in her blood. Lewis noted that Sacagawea's pulse was not only weak, but also irregular, and her muscles were twitching. These observations confirm a diminished blood volume and an imbalance of electrolytes. Lewis directed that she be given water from a nearby mineral spring to drink. The journals indicate that the water contained sulfur and almost certainly contained other electrolytes. The water from Giant Springs, a tourist attraction at Great Falls, adjacent to the Missouri River and not far from the spring that Sacagawea drank from, has been carefully analyzed. Water from Giant Springs is significantly alkaline and contains high enough concentrations of sodium (11 miligrams/liter), potassium (2 miligrams/liter), and calcium (86 miligrams/liter) to correct any electrolyte disturbance caused by dehydration. The high concentration of calcium would have been particularly beneficial in stopping her muscle twitching. The spring that supplied water for Sacagawea may not have had the identical mineral content, but it is close enough geographically to make a similar analysis likely.

Sacagawea was sick for a week and convalescent for two or three days before she recovered completely and was able to proceed with the portage past the Great Falls. Unfortunately, she indulged in the "white apples," an edible root also known as the prairie apple, and had a recurrence of abdominal pain. Lewis blamed Charbonneau—who by this time was likely to be blamed by Lewis for almost anything that went wrong—for allowing her to eat forbidden food. He said that if Sacagawea died it would be Charbonneau's fault. All returned to normal, however, and she made a complete recovery. The reason for her cure may not have been understood, but it was certainly fortuitous. This illness came at both a fortunate and a critical moment. Fortunate because they were camped for a few days and preparing to make a portage around the falls, and critical because there might have been a serious delay if she had not recovered enough to walk the 18-mile portage. Her illness never recurred. If Sacagawea had died the expedition would have proceeded, but the men might have run into serious difficulties when they met the Shoshones. They would not have had an interpreter for the vital task of acquiring horses. In addition, as a woman, Sacagawea was a token of peace in the group: evidence to other Indians that the Corps was not a war party. Baptiste would almost certainly have died soon after his mother. He was only four months old and totally dependent on Sacagawea for food and care. The men of the expedition would undoubtedly have tried to feed the infant, but they had no substitute for breast milk, and there were no other Indians nearby to whom they could have given the child.

The expedition now embarked on the most exhausting, stressful weeks of the entire voyage. Perhaps it was fortunate that they did not know how far they had to struggle to reach a navigable river on the Western Slope. If they had foreseen the hardships they would have to withstand for the next few weeks there might have been some grumblings and indecision about going farther. The snow-covered mountains told a story they did not really want to hear.

The next important stage was to portage around the falls. Some of the men reconnoitered a route and marked it with stakes, while the others prepared makeshift wagons to carry the canoes and equipment. The route was rough and covered with prickly pear cactus. The men's moccasins were thin, and the cactus spines penetrated their feet. The mosquitoes and gnats were pestilential and deerflies added to the misery. The weather was hot, except for the strong summer rains that brought hailstones as big as apples. The wagon axles broke and had to be repaired. At rests along the way the men fell into exhausted sleep. This was, perhaps, the supreme physical effort of the whole expedition. The portage started on June 22 and finished twelve days later.

While the men were hauling and pushing the heavy wagons, Lewis was at the upper camp trying to assemble the iron boat he had spent so much time designing at Harper's Ferry and which they had carried all the way from Pittsburgh. There were unforeseeable problems. They did not have enough animals for the skins because the buffalo had moved on. Then they sewed the skins with sharp, triangular cutting needles that made holes in the hides that were difficult to seal. Finally, they were in an area without any fir trees, and without firs there was no resin, and without resin there was no good seal for the seams. Lewis improvised a sealant of grease and coals that looked fine. The boat floated well for a time, settled in the water, and then water began pouring in through every seam. "The evil was irreparable," he wrote, "I therefore relinquished all hope of my favorite boat and ordered her to be sunk in the water."

The failure of the frame boat presented another crisis. The Corps needed canoes to carry the men up the river. The hunters reported that there were larger trees upstream. Lady Luck smiled again. Big trees were found, and the canoes were built. Their transportation was gradually diminishing. They had started with a large keelboat and two pirogues. After the winter they were reduced to one pirogue and several smaller canoes, and now they would have only two canoes.

During this period York became sick with a fever that Lewis treated with tartar emetic, and he recovered quickly. Clark, however, had a febrile illness for several days. It was not a recurrent fever and he did not report that he had a rash, but he possibly had tick fever. Ticks were abundant; it was the right season of the year, and nowadays, tick fever is endemic in this area. He too recovered.

Ticks are the vectors for several diseases: Rocky Mountain spotted fever and Colorado tick fever would both have been possible, but Colorado tick fever would have been the more likely. It starts with a high fever, headache, and general feeling of illness. In about half the cases the fever lasts two to three days, disappears, and returns a couple of days later. In a few cases there is an accompanying rash. Clark had the fever and general illness of sufficient severity to make tick fever likely. He did not have a rash and the fever did not recur, but the absence of these features would not rule out the disease. Whatever he had, it was almost certainly not malaria.

A third tick-associated problem would have been disastrous, tick paralysis. The victim is bitten by a tick, often on the back of the neck. Over a number of days the person becomes progressively paralyzed and can die from generalized failure of the respiratory muscles. The cure is miraculous and simple. Remove the tick. This disease was first recognized at the beginning of the twentieth century by a veterinarian who was asked to see paralyzed sheep. He found engorged ticks on their skin, and they recovered when the ticks were removed. If this had happened to a member of the expedition he would almost certainly have died unless the tick had been found and removed.

After the new canoes had been built the expedition moved upstream, soon coming to the Three Forks that the Captains named the Jefferson, Madison, and Gallatin, not being willing to pick out one as the Missouri. They chose to ascend the Jefferson and made the correct choice. They were coming into the country of the Shoshones and camped on the exact spot where Sacagawea had been captured by the Hidatsa war party. Lewis could not tell if Sacagawea was glad to be back or sad at the recollection of her capture and imprisonment. She told the officers that the expedition was entering the summer territory of her tribe. Signs of Indians increased and Lewis, like Robinson Crusoe, found a fresh footprint in the sand that he knew to be Indian because the large toe turned inward. Perhaps the print belonged to a scout who had discovered them and run away in alarm.

The story of Lewis meeting the Shoshones is one of the most dramatic turning points in American history. The Corps had come this far and was searching for the tribe they hoped would help them. The first sighting was of a scout on a horse, dark against the sky. Lewis made what he thought were the universal signs of friendship and laid down his gun while bringing out beads and other gifts. The scout, who was mounted bareback on an "elegant" horse, allowed Lewis to approach to within 100 yards when he suddenly turned his horse around, gave it a whack with his whip, jumped the stream, and was gone. Lewis' frustration was turned against the men with him, for he thought their behavior had frightened the Indian.

Two days later Lewis came upon an old Indian woman and two girls. At first, they thought he was about to kill them and bowed in submission to their fate. He persuaded them he was friendly, gave them gifts, and asked to be taken to their village. One of the girls had fled, and soon a war party of sixty Indians came galloping up ready to do battle. But the old woman pacified them and soon suspicion had turned to friendship. The signs of friendship were so effusive with hugging and rubbing of cheeks that Lewis would have been glad if their welcome had come to a halt.

Lewis and his men were ahead of the main party, and he had to persuade the Indians that others were coming behind him who were equally friendly. The Indians were naturally suspicious, and it was only through a masterpiece of diplomacy and trust that trouble was avoided. Eventually the others arrived. It had been a long and difficult haul over the rocky streambed. They were also greeted effusively, especially when the Indians saw a woman in the party, a sign that the group came in peace. The emotional climax, a climax so unlikely that most novelists would be laughed at for including it in a story, came when Sacagawea realized that the Shoshone Chief, Cameawhait, was her brother. Even Lewis had to admit that "the meeting of those people was really affecting."

The Indians were desperately poor and lived on the edge of starvation. When word came that one of the hunters had shot a deer the men ran to the carcass and began to tear at the raw flesh and eat the intestines with feces and gastric juice dribbling from the corners of their mouths. Lewis was horrified and disgusted by this display of animal hunger but recognized the state of privation in which they lived.

The reunited Corps made preparations for the next stage. Clark was sent to explore a possible river, although the Indians said that it was impossible to navigate. It was. It was the River of No Return, the upper reaches of the Snake that plunge and twist through canyons that would have been a death trap for the clumsy canoes they were going to make. The only alternative was to go through the mountains on foot and horse and reach a navigable river. Cameawhait sold them horses, although the tribe was short of horses following a Hidatsa raid in the spring. An old man they called Toby agreed to guide them through the mountains.

One day, while going with the group to the upper Shoshone camp, Lewis noticed that one of the Indian women gave her duties to another woman and disappeared. He asked what had happened and was told, nonchalantly, that the woman had stepped off the trail to give birth and would be rejoining them shortly. True enough, an hour later, the woman appeared with a newborn infant strapped to her back. The apparent casualness with which the Indians regarded childbirth amazed Lewis. A theory existed that the Indian women had easy labor because they were used to carrying heavy loads on their backs. But, as Lewis pointed out, the Shoshone women were not in the habit of carrying loads but used horses to carry them, yet still had no problems with childbirth. It was reported that Indian women who had children fathered by white men had much more difficulty in labor. No explanation was offered, but it might be that the offspring of white men were larger than those fathered by Indians, and Sacagawea, bearing her first child, fathered by a white man, had a difficult labor.

The expedition set out from the Shoshone Camp on August 26, 1805. They had twenty-nine horses to carry loads, and, although not every man rode, Sacagawea and her son were given a horse.

When the group started, Lewis was riding but gave his horse to one of the men who was sick and unable to walk. During the next month the men had a living as lean as that of the Indians. Game was in very short supply. There were days when the hunters shot nothing except a couple of spruce grouse. Analyzing what was available to eat, day by day, the tally is small: four salmon; seven deer; three deer; one deer, one goose, one grouse; four salmon, one deer; nothing but berries. Slim pickings for more than thirty people exerting themselves to the maximum.

The route through the mountains and forests was hard. Sometimes there was a trail, at other times the men had to bushwhack through the forest, clambering over fallen trees. They went along steep canyons. Horses fell from the trail or were injured in the fallen timber. The weather turned cold with snow and rain. They were wet, and Clark was afraid he was going to freeze his feet (which had been frozen twice before). When food was in too short supply they killed a horse or a colt. Lewis broke out the portable soup, a nutritious but unpalatable substitute for fresh venison or buffalo. Salmon was not the favorite food of the men who were used to meat, and the crushed roots and berries they obtained from the Indians did not satisfy them.

There is a saying that you can live three minutes without oxygen, three days without water, and three weeks without food. During the month it took for the Corps to get through the mountains there were days when they had very little food. They were hungry, but not starving. After killing a colt Lewis wrote that they "supped on it heartily and thought it very fine meat."

The men's health began to deteriorate. Boils and dysentery became a problem, and, even after they came out of the mountains and met the Nez Percé Indians on September 20, their troubles were not over. (The Nez Percé were also called the Chopunnish.) The relief at finding themselves off the hellish trail through the mountains and on flatland again was tempered by an epidemic of dysentery that flattened almost everyone in the group. As soon as they began to eat food they had bought from the Indians they became sick. Was it the food? Was it this change of diet to dried fish and roots and berries? Or was it an intestinal infection that swept through the camp? The most likely medical explanation is that it was infectious gastroenteritis attacking a group of men already weakened by a month of minimal rations and extreme effort. They took a long time to recover. Lewis was particularly affected and, going from one Indian camp to another, could barely ride "on a gentle horse." It must have been depressing and humiliating for a Virginian gentleman, used to riding the finest horses, to barely be able to stay in the saddle of a quiet Indian nag. Time and doses of Rush's pills cleaned out the infection, and, slowly, the men began to recover and regain enough strength to cut down trees and make canoes for the final stage to the coast. The Indians were generous and helpful. They told the Corps what to expect on the downstream journey and offered to act as guides and go-betweens with the downstream tribes. They agreed to look after the horses until the expedition returned in the spring. A few days into October 1805 the Corps loaded their new canoes and headed downstream, a welcome relief from the toil of upstream travel. They were entering a new world, not always a world of plenty, and certainly one with different weather. Their diet also changed. They ate salmon and added dogs to their menu. Most of the men liked dog meat, but Clark never brought himself to savor it.

When the expedition entered the Columbia they found a population of Indian tribes that relied on fishing and trade for their living. The Columbia also had falls and rapids that had to be portaged, and, once, the Corps ran a rapid that the Indians did not think they could survive. The nonswimmers were made to walk, and the others roller-coasted down the river, avoiding rocks and holes, and made it safely through. All these rapids have been flooded by the water that now rises behind the Bonneville Dam, east of Portland. What was once a wild, uncontrolled river, whose level rose and fell with flow from rainstorms and melting snow, is now benign and broad. The millions of chinook salmon that ran the river when Lewis passed this way are now reduced to an annual migration of only three hundred thousand, all carefully counted as they swim past a window in the side of the fish run. The wealth of the river has changed from salmon to electricity.

The expedition finally sailed on to the broad delta of the river, and on November 5, Clark wrote in his journal, "Ocian in view! O! the Joy." Two days later they could hear the sea, "and the roreing or noise made by the waves braking on the rocky shores." They pulled into a narrow inlet near the modern village of Skamokawa (named after the man who was Chief at the time of Lewis and Clark) where they traded with the Indians for fish, giving small gifts, handkerchiefs, beads, and trinkets. The river was wide and smooth, but already the explorers knew that they were in tidal waters. Gulls flew overhead and the waters rose and fell every day. They were close to their goal of the Pacific.

The Chinook Indians who lived along both shores of the western reaches of the Columbia were an ancient tribe with a strong civilization, established villages, and a mythology that told them they had come from the Far North. They had already had some contact with white men. In 1792, Captain Robert Gray, an American sea Captain, had sent a party ashore up what is now the Gray River and had named the main river Columbia, after his ship the *Columbia Rediviva*. Even earlier, around 1780, a red-haired white man, Jack Ramsay, who had been shipwrecked and landed on the shore, had lived with the Indians farther down the coast and had fathered two sons, one of whom was described on several occasions as a frecklefaced, red-headed Indian who seemed to understand but could not speak English.

In 1781 and 1782, smallpox swept through the tribe leaving behind a trail of sorrow. The terrible disease that left pockmarked faces was seen as a disgrace, and those who survived were shunned. Villages were abandoned and the dead hung from the trees, mute evidence of the destruction the disease had brought. The Indians were terrified by this introduction to the white man's civilization. In 1845, the historian John Dunn recorded the frantic efforts of the Indians to cure the disease and halt the smallpox epidemic. The charms and potions of their shamans were to no avail. Those who became infected were abandoned and left to die. Some who escaped the attack fled. Others committed suicide, despondent, hopeless, or shamed by the ugliness of their pockmarked faces. Some tribes were completely destroyed.

Five miles east of present-day Skamokawa, Washington, two narrow branches of the river surround a small island, thick with old-growth Sitka spruce, the larger trees more than four hundred years old. These ancient trees managed to escape the saws of the lumbermen a century ago because they were inaccessible; now they stand as silent memorials to the Lewis and Clark expedition.

On November 7, 1805, Clark wrote:

> We set out . . . the fog so thick we could not See across the river, two Canos of Indians met and returned with us to their village which is Situated behind a cluster of Marshey islands, in a narrow channel . . . through which we passed to the village of 4 Houses, they gave us to eat some fish and Sold us, fish, *Wap pa to* roots and three dogs and 2 otter skins for which we gave fish hooks principally of which they were verry fond . . . about 14 miles below . . . we landed at a village of the same form of those above, here we purchased a dog, some fish, *Wa pa to* and I purchased 2 beaver skins for the purpose of making me a roab, as the robe I have is roten and good for nothing . . . we proceeded on about 12 miles and encamped under a high hill . . . opposite to a rock situated half a mile from the shore, about 50 feet high and 20 feet in diameter . . . great joy in camp we are in view of the Ocian, this great Pacific ocean which we have been so long anxious to see.

The Corps camped close to the sea, the rain falling in sheets and the waves crashing against the shore, piling huge logs against the rocks on which they had set up a shelter. It was a wet, miserable place, and they knew they could not spend the winter there. Their clothes were wet and rotting, and Clark thought it was lucky that the weather was not too cold. If they did not have an opportunity to make new clothes before the winter they would "suffer very much." Unknowingly, they were prime candidates for hypothermia and immersion foot, a condition caused by exposure of the legs for several days to cold wetness.

Local Indian women visited "for the purpose of gratifying the passions of our men." Clark thought that the women chased the men openly. Many of the women were good-looking and, to them, there was nothing unseemly about making sexual advances. There was obvious clinical evidence of venereal disease in many of the women and men, but the assignations were clearly not discouraged by the Captains who provided the men with ribbon to "bestow on their favorite lasses." Both the men and the Captains lived to regret these contacts, for many of the men developed gonorrhea and later were implored by their officers to abstain and avoid more disease.

The rain and wind continued, confining the men to their camp, wet, and uncomfortable. Indians visited the camp and sold them *wappato,* a plant they had not eaten before. This root, better known as arrowhead, was a common item for trade between the Indians and became a staple of the Corps' diet during the next months. It is still found in the low ground around the Columbia River. An island off the south shore of the river, Sauvie Island, was, at the time of the expedition called *Wappato* Island because of the abundance of the bulbs that grew there. Now, it is a quiet farming haven and a wildlife refuge where Canada geese and sandhill cranes winter in the tens of thousands.

The Indians said that game was abundant on the southern shore, and the group had a long discussions about where to spend the winter. The advantage of staying on the north shore would be a greater likelihood of meeting with a foreign trading vessel. But there was little shelter on the northern coast, exposed to the winter southwesterlies, and game seemed to be scarce. A vote was taken, a vote that has assumed historical significance because both a woman, Sacagawea, and a slave, York, were allowed to vote. Twenty-five voted to cross to the south side and find a suitable place. Sacagawea was not listed with those who voted, but Clark added a sentence, "Janey in favor of a place where there is plenty of potas." "Janey" was a nickname given Sacagawea by Clark.

The Corps returned upstream, afraid of making the crossing to where Astoria now stands. The river was too wide, the currents and tide too strong, and the waves too high. The Indians, in their beautiful high-prowed canoes had no trouble and no fear, but the heavy canoes of the Corps would have capsized and sunk. They went upstream for several miles and crossed safely on November 26, 1805.

When Lewis went searching for a place to build their winter home he demanded certain criteria: enough game for food, wood for building huts and fuel, water for drinking, reasonable access to the ocean where they would obtain salt, not too close to an Indian village, high enough to avoid spring tides, and accessible by canoe. In December the men started to cut the trees, split and trim the logs, and build the cabins for a new winter home. They named the place Fort Clatsop after the local Indian tribe.

From the time they started downstream, high in the mountains, until they landed near the site of what would become Fort Clatsop, there were hardly any entries in the journals about illnesses or accidents. Perhaps the thrill of moving downstream and the thought of reaching the ocean, the objective of their dreams, overcame their concern for minor complaints. The expedition had overcome tremendous difficulties and odds. The journey had been longer and more perilous than they had anticipated. When they got home they would have a few things to say to the armchair geographers about the "short" portage between one river and another. They would also have plenty to say about the size of the mountains that had snow-covered peaks in the middle of summer. They would have wonders to describe that many people would not believe. But, at last, they had reached the ocean. Perhaps a ship would sail into the mouth of the Columbia bringing traders, and perhaps some of the Corps would be able to sail home instead of crossing the mountains again. For the moment, on Christmas day 1805, they were under shelter, with a fire to keep them warm, and a roof over their heads. They could look forward to the next Christmas in their own homes, 3,000 miles away.

SEVEN

Rain, Fleas, and Thoughts of Home: December 1805–March 1806

L ife at Fort Clatsop was not fun. In the 106 days the Corps spent there the weather was fair on only twelve, and the sun shone on only six. There was a small amount of snow, but the chief misery was almost constant rain. Elk-skin clothes rotted, and colds, sniffles, and rheumatism were the order of the day. Hunting in a wet forest with water dripping from every tree and bush must have been a thankless task. The men were discovering the miseries of a soggy Northwest Coast winter. Historian James Ronda of the University of Tulsa described the situation well, "A season at Fort Clatsop seemed to promise mildew, spoiled meat and numbing boredom." He might have added the unremitting plague of fleas that inhabited every Indian home and soon invaded the huts where the men lived, infesting their clothing and becoming a daily nuisance. The men spent hours picking the unwelcome visitors out of blankets and the seams of clothes.

Clark drew a plan of Fort Clatsop in his diary: two rows of rooms facing each other, three on one side and four on the other. The whole fort was only 50 feet square and surrounded by a sharp, pointed picket fence. Between the rows of buildings was an open space, called by some a parade ground, although only a minuscule parade could have been held there. A gate at one end of the open space gave access to the fort and was closed at night to keep out the Indians. The men lived in the three huts on one side; on the other, Charbonneau, Sacagawea, and Baptiste occupied one room, Lewis and Clark the next, York and another man the third, and the fourth room was a storage place for meat.

One of the immediate tasks was to distill salt from the sea, so Clark found a suitable place 15 miles southwest of the fort near a long beach, now the site of the town of Seaside, Oregon. In order to be able to distill the maximum amount of salt from the water, pure seawater had to be used. It would have been easier and quicker to go the 4 miles to the shore close by, but there the water would have been diluted with freshwater from the Columbia River as it spilled out of the estuary and down the coast. The longer route was difficult, but essential. The way was not easy, through thick forest, across rivers and sloughs, and was made more difficult by the need to carry the heavy metal kettles in which the water would be boiled.

A reproduction of the Corps' fireplace has been built at the foot of a quiet residential street in Seaside: a pile of stones long enough

---

The National Park Service has built an exact replica of Fort Clatsop according to Clark's plans. The buildings stand on a slight rise, high enough to be above any high tides, and a hundred yards from the Netul River. A path leads from the camp to the river where a replica of a canoe lies in the grass a few yards from the water. I visited Fort Clatsop, 195 years, almost to the day, after the expedition headed for home, and rain was falling gently from a leaden sky. In all the years, the weather had not changed much. There were no other visitors, and I stood back at the edge of the clearing, with my eyes shut, imagining the sights and sounds of the camp: men coming in from hunting, wood being chopped for the fires, Indians gathering around the gate, anxious to trade and sell their roots and pounded salmon. The smell of smoke drifted across through the trees, and somewhere, a small child was crying like the spirit of Baptiste.

---

to support five kettles, with holes underneath each kettle, and a space underneath for the fire. The high-tide mark is only 100 yards away, separated from the salt camp by low dunes. High tide may have been closer two hundred years ago because, over time, the beach has been filling in. North of the camp the beach stretches for more than a mile. To the south looms the dark, tree-covered mass of Tillamook Head. Gulls wheel overhead, and flocks of sanderlings race on invisible, speeding legs along the advancing tide, rising with nervous energy, to land again farther down the beach.

A small Tillamook Indian village with friendly, impoverished occupants was situated nearby. It was an occasional source of food for the small salt camp, although the Indians lived mostly off fish they found washed up on the shore. The men must have built themselves a shelter, for they stayed there several weeks until they had distilled enough salt to last all the way back to St. Louis. It was an isolated place without any possibility of immediate help. While the salt seekers were there, one man became so sick that he had to be taken back to Fort Clatsop in a litter, and another cut his leg severely. As happened so frequently, the men were left on their own and had to rely on their wits to feed and survive. Some would hunt, while the others kept filling the kettles with seawater, scraping out the salt, and cutting wood for the fires. They were not as comfortable as the men at the fort but were better off than the Indians. They had rifles and could hunt elk for food, but they must have spent many hours standing around the fire, warming themselves, drying their clothes, and spinning yarns.

Life back at the fort soon began to take on a routine. Hunters went out every day, but not all were equally successful. Drewyer was consistently the best hunter, often bringing back an elk—or several—when the others shot nothing. He must have been a consummate artist at moving silently through the forest, sensing the wind, knowing where to find game, and, finally, being able to stalk close enough to take that one fatal shot. The carcasses frequently had to be left many miles from camp, and, by the time they were retrieved, the meat had often spoiled. The men were not living in the natural refrigerator of Fort Mandan, and the combination of a warmer, wetter climate was not conducive to preserving meat.

As the winter progressed the hunting became more difficult. The elk herds that lived nearby became depleted and the survivors moved away. By the beginning of March 1806, Lewis wrote that "the elk had all gone off to the mountains a considerable distance from us. This is unwelcome information and reather allarming we have only two days provision on hand, and that nearly spoiled." Part of this disappearance would have been the normal migration of elk from the low winter feeding grounds to the summer's higher breeding territory.

The diet was monotonous—elk meat, roots and berries bought from the Indians, and pounded dried salmon. Occasionally they had a feast. On February 7, 1806, Lewis was able to report: "This evening we had what I call an excellent supper it consisted of a marrowbone piece and a brisket of boiled Elk that had the appearance of a little fat on it. This for Fort Clatsop is living in high style." Fat was always at a premium. The game that was shot was naturally low in fat, and even lower in fat than normal because the animals were in the middle of the privations of winter.

Whale blubber was the fattiest food they ate, and they only ate it twice. Once near the start of their stay at the fort, the Indians brought them a small quantity of blubber. A few days later Willard and Peter Weiser, who had been setting up the salt camp, returned with some blubber obtained from the same whale that had been washed up on the shore. Lewis thought it was white and similar to the fat of pork but "Spungey and Somewhat coarser." He thought its taste resembled beaver or dog, neither of which resonate with a modern reader. The blubber was soon consumed.

The episode of the whale was more than a search for food. Word had come to the camp about a whale on the shore south of the salt camp, and Clark prepared to go there, hoping to acquire a large quantity of whale meat. Sacagawea insisted that she be taken to see the whale and the sea. She argued that she had come all the way from the Missouri River and was not going to be denied the opportunity of seeing both the sea and the whale. So, strapping Baptiste to her back, she joined the party to the salt camp. At the salt camp they hired an Indian guide, for the price of a file, to take them over Tillamook Head to the beach (now Cannon Beach) where the whale was stranded.

Tillamook Head, a forest-covered eminence, dominates the south end of the beach at Seaside. It was a formidable barrier to cross: steep, slippery, and precipitous. The party walked 2.5 miles along the beach to the foot of the climb, where the guide pointed upward and uttered the Indian word for "bad." At first glance the route seemed to Clark to be almost perpendicular, and the summit was shrouded in cloud. It took them two hours of "labour and fatigue" to reach the top from which they could look down on the beach with its rocky offshore sentinels: a beach that is now photographed as the epitome of the rugged Oregon coastline.

The climb over Tillamook Head was a remarkable tribute to the strength and determination of Sacagawea. The idea of scrambling and pulling yourself several hundred feet up a near vertical, rain-sodden hillside with a baby strapped to your back would make the most enthusiastic mountaineer think twice. By the time the party reached the whale, it was only a skeleton 105 feet long, stripped clean of meat. With some difficulty they persuaded the Indians to sell them 120 pounds of blubber to render into oil.

That evening, in camp, a shout of alarm went up. Clark soon discovered that Hugh McNeal, a consistent rogue who was always picking up another dose of venereal disease, was in trouble again. He had been enticed to the hut of one of the Indians with the offer of a woman, but the real intent had been to kill him for his blanket. One of the women had tried, unsuccessfully, to stop McNeal, and when she became aware of the plot started screaming. The Indian responsible was from a distant village, and the locals rallied around to protect the visitors, and even slept at Clark's feet.

The next day Clark was worried that he was so weak from lack of food that he would not be able to climb back over Tillamook Head. He summoned up his energy, however, and from the summit "beheld the grandest and most pleasing prospects which my eyes ever surveyed, in my front the boundless ocean; to the N. and N.E. the coast as far as my sight could be extended, the seas raging with emence waves and brakeing with great force from the rocks of Cape Diapointment to the N.W." The paths along the cliffs of Ecola Park now make the same magnificent view easier to obtain. Offshore, black sea stacks, streaked with guano, and home to tens of thousands of seabirds called murres, jut from the waves. The way down to the salt camp was no easier than the climb up. They met a group of Indians carrying heavy loads. Clark found one Indian woman, about to fall down the precipitous slope, holding a 100-pound load by a single strap, and hanging on to a bush with the other hand. He tried to support her load but could barely lift it; then her husband came to the rescue. They arrived back at the salt camp so fatigued that Clark insisted they stay until the next morning before returning to the fort.

Most of the men greatly favored salt with their meat, but to Clark it was a matter of total indifference. Regardless of taste, having enough salt in the diet was essential to men who expended as much physical effort as they did. During the cool of the winter the need for salt was not as great as during the summer when the salt lost in sweat was considerable. Eventually, by the end of February 1806, they had made about 20 gallons of salt, more than enough to last them back to Missouri, and they abandoned the salt camp. Salt, while enhancing the taste of food, is an essential component of the human body and necessary for the normal function of every cell.

Lewis hardly ever left the camp during the many weeks the expedition stayed at Fort Clatsop. He spent long hours writing in his journal. It was as though he was making up for the many days he had written nothing and had relied on Clark for the nitty-gritty details of their progress. Frequently Lewis and Clark wrote identical accounts in their respective journals, duplicating the entries in case one journal was lost. Clark also wrote long accounts, and writing was clearly one way to overcome the boredom of their stay. They were not exploring new territory, meeting new Indians, fighting, or struggling for their lives. Their existence was relatively benign. Discipline and trade with the Indians had to be maintained, but when the journal entries began with "No occurrence worthy of relation took place today," or, "Nothing worthy of notice occurred today," it is obvious that they were searching for more excitement.

Relations with the local Indians were very different from those they had experienced at Fort Mandan. There, the Indians had been a close and integral part of their lives, and the traffic between the Mandan villages and the fort was steady and at times, intimate. The Captains were learning about what lay in store for them and spoke to anyone who could give them information about the route through the mountains and the ocean. A similar rapport between the men and the Chinook Indians never blossomed at Fort Clatsop.

The Mandans and Hidatsas were the type of Indians the Corps was used to: tall, lean, warlike, and sometimes aggressive. The Plains Indians grew crops and rode horses, and they had some conception of a Great Father in Washington and the possibilities of future trade. They could be called "My Children" and accepted the patronizing relationship with apparent grace. Not so at Fort Clatsop. The physical appearance of the West Coast Indians, particularly the Clatsops, was different and foreign. Both Lewis and Clark thought the natives were "illy formed"—short, stocky, with broader faces and flattened heads. Their clothes hid little below the waist, they squatted like frogs, and the women tied bands around their legs that made their ankles swell. They did not fight with their neighbors, preferring the give-and-take of trade to raiding and scalping. They had been trading for years with English and American merchants who sailed up the Columbia and stayed for several months of business. They were sharp bargainers who knew well how to leave the table and return the next day and continue haggling over prices. They knew that, above all, the white men wanted otter skins, and they must have been quickly disappointed that this new group of white men had nothing to trade but trinkets, and did not even seem interested in trade beyond their immediate needs.

The Clatsop Indians, the tribe that lived near the fort, were a subgroup of the Chinooks. Their appearance may have been different from that of the Plains Indians, and even unpleasant to the men of the Corps, but they were a sophisticated tribe with great skills in weaving and the building of elegant, seaworthy canoes. Their plank houses, which have been compared with the Vikings' halls, were large and accommodated several families. With the planks of the wall securely buried 3 to 5 feet into the ground, the structures were solid, warm, and weatherproof. These were not the temporary dwellings of nomads but the permanent homes of a fixed people.

It is difficult to understand the antipathy that seemed to be immediate between Lewis and the Clatsops. He thought they were thieves and regarded them as a threat. Soon after the fort was built Lewis promulgated orders that ensured that Indians could not stay overnight in the fort and could only be allowed within the walls after the Sergeant of the Guard had been informed of their presence. At the end of the day even the most important visitors were unceremoniously shown the door. The Indians, for their part, never showed the slightest intent to harm anyone. They came to trade and to find out what this new group wanted and had to offer. It soon became obvious that the visitors did not want much and had little to offer. The Clatsops had no concept of the distance between them and Washington, and Lewis never made any "My Children" speeches to them. The Louisiana Purchase had only given the United States jurisdiction as far as the Rockies, so the fort was in a political never-never land. The British rivals, however, were not a constant presence and had only been trading along the West Coast since 1792, when Lieutenant Broughton sailed up the Columbia. Lewis had neither the right nor the inclination to suggest that if the Indians played the game right, they would be rewarded with protection and trading posts.

In his journal Lewis described the artifacts of Indian life in great detail: houses, pots and cooking, clothes and waterproof hats, weapons, arrows, paddles, and canoes. He was particularly intrigued and impressed by their beautiful canoes that were lighter, could carry larger loads, and were more manageable than the rough canoes the Corps had built. Because of the lack of communication between the Indians and Lewis and Clark—in part because none of the Corps could speak their language—the journals concentrate more on the details of life than the culture and beliefs of the people. The names of the tribes were listed, as were the number of houses they inhabited and their populations. The journals contained few references to their diseases, and, in contrast to the experience earlier and later in the voyage, the Indians seldom asked for medical attention in return for goods or services.

From a medical and sociological standpoint the most interesting habit of the Clatsop and Chinook Indians was the way they flattened the heads of their infants. Soon after birth the infant was strapped to a board, and a second board, attached by a hinge to the top of the first, was pressed down on the forehead, flattening the face from the tip of the nose to the crown of the head. Not only was this appearance regarded as a sign of beauty, but it was also a sign that the person was free and not a slave. To have a "round head" was the sign of servitude, the mark of a slave. Although Lewis and Clark never commented on this in their journals, the Indians must have wondered why all the white men were slaves. The habit now seems abhorrent to us, but white observers at the time said that the appearance was not distasteful, and there is no evidence that the development or intellect of the child was adversely affected.

The expedition had been profligate in giving away gifts and rewards in the earlier part of the trip and now had pathetically small amounts of trading goods. "Two handkerchiefs would now contain all the small articles of merchandize which we now possess; the balance of the stock consist of 6 blue robes one scarlet do, one uniform artillerist's coat and hat, five robes made of our large flag, and a few old cloaths trimmed with ribbon"—scant supplies for trade and exchange all the way back across the mountains. The strangest gift was a pair of satin breeches given to a local Chief. Lewis—and perhaps the Chief—obviously regarded this gift as one of great value, but it conjures up the almost absurd picture of an

Indian, used to wearing nothing below his waist, walking around in satin. A less practical material for the environment would be hard to imagine.

Sometimes the gifts were not enough to purchase what the men needed. Before leaving Fort Clatsop Lewis wanted to buy an Indian canoe. Sergeant Pryor had purchased a canoe in exchange for Lewis' laced coat and some tobacco, but they still needed another. The Clatsops would not sell one at a price they could afford. The Indians valued their canoes second only to their wives, so, to the discredit of the Corps, four men stole a canoe from the Clatsops and hid it so that the crime would not be detected. Lewis consoled his conscience by saying that the canoe was in return for some elk carcasses the Indians had purloined, even though three dogs, for eating, had been offered in compensation for the elk. This robbery was the single greatest blot on the behavior of the Corps during all the years of the expedition, one that could not be explained away by a slim excuse.

In spite of the Corps' generally cool feelings toward the Indians, there were times when relations between the two groups were cordial. At the time of their departure to return to the East, Lewis gave Chief Comowooll, one of the local Clatsop Chiefs, a certificate of good conduct in recognition of "the friendly intercourse which he has maintained with us during our residence at this place."

If there was little mention of illness among the Indians, there was a steady stream of illness among the men of the expedition. On February 10, 1806, Willard arrived back from the salt camp with a badly cut knee. He had shot an elk and, while butchering it with his tomahawk, slashed his knee. He returned to the fort as he could not continue to make salt. When he returned he reported that Bratton and Gibson were also sick. Gibson was so sick with a fever that he could not stand. Sergeant Pryor and four other men took Gibson back to the fort. Strong winds prevented them from finding a safe place to get Gibson across the river that runs parallel to the shore. By the time the party reached the fort, Gibson was feeling better and was not as ill as expected. He still had a fever but was not in any danger. He was treated with niter and sage tea, and his feet were bathed in warm water. At night he was given thirty-nine drops of laudanum, a good dose that would have made him sleepy and contented.

Bratton was described as being "much reduced" but seemed to be recovering fast. His apparent recovery was temporary, and for the next two months he had a series of problems, the most serious of which was severe back pain that made it impossible for him to work, and at times, even to walk. When the Corps left Fort Clatsop in March Bratton was still sick, without any signs of recovery. His illness turned out to be the longest of any during the expedition.

Bratton's back pain became worse, and Lewis gave him Peruvian bark and saltpeter to break his fever. However, his fever persisted, so he was given a dose of Rush's pills that Lewis had found to be efficacious for patients with boils. In the evening his fever abated and he felt better. A day later he was given more bark, as was Gibson, who had improved more than his friend. Lewis thought that Gibson would recover, but expressed no opinion about Bratton. He was concerned and worried about any man who did not recover quickly in response to treatment. If the man did not respond to Rush's pills and Peruvian bark there were not many other therapeutic options. (Most of Lewis' journal entry that day was a detailed description of the California condor.)

Two days later Lewis wrote of Bratton, "He is very weak and complains of his back." He was given six Scott's pills. There is no record of Scott's pills in the medical kit, and while there is uncertainty about their properties it can be assumed that they were laxatives rather than analgesics. They had no effect, and as six of them were given without any result they cannot have been very powerful or were of uncertain potency. During the winter at Fort Clatsop someone was sick almost every day. If the problem was not with Bratton or Gibson, another man was sick. By February 20, Gibson was improving rapidly, but Bratton was no better. In fact, he seemed to be worse. And McNeal, who had developed syphilis earlier, was also becoming worse, probably due to inattention to treatment. He had been one of the men at the salt camp and, without supervision, may have been lax in continuing his treatment. His name came up several times because of his repeated attacks of venereal disease. He was too fond of the "tawny damsels" for his own good. Willard joined the sick parade with a headache and loss of appetite.

Scott's pills were administered to Willard and Bratton but only worked for Willard. Gibson, still not better, received Peruvian bark three times a day and improved. By February 22, the number of men on sick call had increased to five: Bratton, Gibson, McNeal, Ordway, and Willard. There had not been as many men sick on the same day since they had left the Wood River Camp two years before. They were suffering from bad colds and fevers, "something I believe of the influenza." Fortunately, all seemed to be improving.

The course of the mini-epidemic varied from day to day. On the twenty-third, Ordway was the sickest and the others were better. On the twenty-fourth, all were improving, and Lewis devoted most of the space in his journal to a description of candlefish, the eulachon, which had arrived in the ocean a few miles away. Millions of these fish, about 10 inches long, migrate up the rivers of the Northwest in the spring and can be easily caught in nets. They are called candlefish because they are so fat that a string drawn through the body can be lit and act as a wick. Lewis found them best to eat when cooked Indian style, roasted together on a spit. Their fat made other preparation unnecessary. Lewis thought they were superior in taste to any fish he had ever eaten, "even more delicate and luscious than the white fish of the lakes."

Willard worsened, but then improved. On March 2, Lewis opened his journal by writing that the diet was so poor that the invalids recovered their strength slowly. But by then none of the men was sick and all had good appetites, although they only had lean elk to eat. Later that day Drewyer arrived back at the fort with a good supply of candlefish and *wappato*. Presumably, the diet improved for a few days. A day later Jean Baptiste LePage was sick and was given Scott's pills, which, again, did not work.

The men were living in very close quarters, and it is not surprising that if one became sick with a viral infection the others would soon catch the same infection. The climate, poor diet, and constantly wet clothes were not the causes of the illnesses but did not help the men to resist whatever infection was spreading in the huts. The diet may have been monotonous, but the meat was supplemented with berries and roots and dried salmon that the Indians brought. The occasional addition of a delicacy such as the candlefish, beaver, whale blubber, or dog helped to broaden the menu and led Lewis to write, "Once more we live in clover; Anchovies fresh sturgeon and Wappatoe." Sometimes the larder was almost empty, with only a couple of days' food in storage; but the men never starved and were never reduced to the same straits they had experienced while coming through the mountains.

The next health problem was an accident, not an illness. A large log fell on Hall's foot and leg. He was lucky that no bones were broken. Bratton relapsed and became sick again, and Lewis still regretted that he could not provide a better diet for the convalescents. A day later the pain in Bratton's back was so severe that he could not rise from his bed. He was given a flannel shirt (only fifteen flannel shirts were brought for the whole group) and his back was bandaged with flannel and rubbed with a liniment made from spirits of wine, camphor, castile soap, and laudanum. That evening he felt better.

Bratton's progress was a seesaw. One day he seemed to be getting better, but the next his back was very painful. March 8 was a good day. Bratton was free of pain and McNeal and Goodrich, two men with syphilis, were told they could stop their mercury treatment. March 9, however, was a bad day for Bratton. Lewis thought "this pain to be something of the rheumatism. We still apply the liniment and flannel: in the evening he was much better." Whatever the underlying cause, Bratton was probably having bad lower back muscle spasms, which were relieved by the liniment and the warm flannel. The treatment gave relief but did not cure the problem.

During this time Lewis wrote a lot about the birds and wildlife: the thousands of snow geese on the beaches; the grebes in the river; the golden and bald eagles; the trout, salmon, and suckers; and the porpoises that came up the river and were sometimes caught by the Indians. He wrote about the way the Indians chased and harpooned whales, although he thought—probably correctly—that more whales died from running afoul of the coast than were killed by the Indians. The descriptions were meticulous and scientific, measuring the size of the salmon (2 to 3 feet long), the arrangement of their teeth, their fins, the taste of the roe, and how the Indians dried the roe in the sun to preserve it for a long time. The Indians told them that the salmon would begin to run early in April. And, anticipating this as a source of food while ascending the river, Lewis determined that they should leave the fort around April 1.

On March 15, the Corps was already making preparations for leaving, and perhaps the rumor had spread to the Indians that the fort would soon be empty and the business opportunities would come to an end. One of the businessmen who decided to pay a visit was Delashshelwit, a Chinook Chief who lived on the northern shore of the Columbia. In November, when the Corps had camped near his village, he and his wife had appeared with some girls with whom the men had sexual relations, several of them catching venereal diseases as a result. Delashshelwit was not going to let another opportunity slip and appeared with his wife, scathingly described by Lewis as "the old baud," and six other women. Lewis did not want another epidemic of venereal disease just as they were about to depart, and he lectured the men and extracted from them a promise that they would not visit the women. Lewis thought that "notwithstanding every effort of their winning graces, the men have preserved their constancy to the vow of celibacy."

The Chief and his entourage stayed near the camp for several days, but eventually left after he was given a certificate of his good deportment and a list of the men who had been at the fort to give to any white trader who visited. These lists of those who had spent the winter at the fort were given to several Indians, in the hope that they would give them to a trader as evidence that the expedition had reached the coast. One of those lists was given to Captain Samuel Hill of Boston on June 12, 1806, but did not reach the States until after the safe return of the expedition to St. Louis. Another reappeared years later and was contemptuously thrown into a fire by the British trader to whom it was given.

Almost on the eve of their departure, Drewyer became ill with severe pain in his side, and was treated by being bled by Clark. Several other men complained of being unwell at the same time. Lewis wrote with typical understatement, "It is truly unfortunate that they should be sick at the moment of our departure." His journal then continued without a pause. "We directed Sgt. Pryor to prepare two canoes. . . ." There was no mention of what would happen if the men did not get well, no suggestion of a contingency plan. Instead, Lewis continued to write long descriptions of Indian clothing and habits, including a description of head flattening. It was as though he was determined to put down every last detail he could think of before the rigors of the return journey made writing difficult or impossible.

The weather did not cooperate. The winds were strong and the rain heavy, delaying the preparations. Many of the men were still ill. Willard and Bratton remained the sickest, and Lewis still thought their illnesses were exacerbated by lack of food. He expected that when they got under way the health of the men would improve. "It has always had that effect on us heretofore." On March 21, Lewis was concerned about Bratton and even wondered if he would recover. His back still hurt and he had pain in his leg and thigh. It is possible that he suffered from a lumbar slipped disc. The characteristic symptom of a slipped intervertebral disc is pain in the back descending into the leg and thigh. Although the problem is in the vertebral column, pain in the leg is due to pressure on nerves that supply the leg. The location of the pain in the leg is precisely related to the nerve root that is compressed, making possible the diagnosis of which disc is involved. In a young, energetic man a slipped or herniated disc was a likely diagnosis, although fever, which accompanied the start of the illness, is not part of the syndrome.

Thoughts and memories of Sergeant Floyd must have been going through Lewis' mind. How would a man as sick as Bratton get up the river and through the mountains? Should he consider leaving him behind in the hope that a ship would soon appear that could take him home? If they left him behind, who would look after him? Lewis did not express such thoughts in his journal, but he and Clark must have discussed them and other possibilities, away from the men, in the quiet of their room. The thought of leaving a man behind would have received short shrift, and all the men departed together.

During the final preparations for departure Lewis recorded his last thoughts on their stay. "Altho' we have not fared sumptuously this winter and spring at Fort Clatsop, we have lived quite as comfortably as we had any reason to expect we should; and have accomplished every object which induced our remaining at this place except that of meeting with the traders who visit the entrance of this river." Even if a ship had come, Lewis would not have allowed any of his men to return on it because he did not want the complement of men depleted. Once again he was thinking of security and the number of men necessary to maintain the strength of the group.

On March 22, a recovered Drewyer and the Fields brothers, Joseph and Reuben, the best hunters, were sent ahead to hunt for the group that would leave the next day. Lewis made some final purchases of food: a dog for the sick men and a small stock of fish. The local Indians reported that several of them had sore throats, and one had died from the disease. Perhaps the Corps was lucky to leave before they were exposed to an epidemic of diphtheria. Lewis' last entry in his journal struck a hopeful note, "The leafing of the huckleberry riminds us of spring."

The Corps of Discovery bade a final adieu to Fort Clatsop at 1:00 P.M. on March 23, 1806, turning their faces toward home with every hope and expectation that the journey would be completed before the leaves of autumn fell.

EIGHT

Back Through the Mountains:
March–September 1806

On the morning of departure from Fort Clatsop the rain was falling in dismal sheets. The Captains wondered if they should delay another day because the weather was so bad, but the sky cleared and the order was given. Go. Even lowering skies and rain could not dampen the enthusiasm as the men loaded the canoes and paddled down the Netul River toward the Columbia. They had only gone a short distance when they met Delashshelwit with the "old baud" and her girls. The Chief still wanted to sell them some fish, a sea-otter skin, and some hats. He was a trader to the last moment, but it was too late for the girls.

The wind was strong as the canoes rounded a point and pushed into the waves of the Columbia. They paddled 16 miles before camping on the shore where Drewyer and Fields, who had gone ahead to hunt for dinner, had set up camp. The hunters had shot two elk, but the carcasses were a couple of miles away, and it was too late to bring them in. That night they did not eat as well as they had hoped. The next morning the group sailed closely along the shore where the waves were not as high and the water was shallow. They stopped at a village and bought *wappato* and a dog to feed the men who were still sick. When they started off down the wrong channel an Indian followed them to set them on the right route and, at the same time, claimed that one of their canoes had been stolen from him. Lewis and his men knew well that one of their canoes had been stolen, but how did the Indian know the story? He may have been correct in his claim, but when he was offered an elk skin in payment, he accepted and turned around without further argument. Both parties were satisfied. Sergeant Ordway was full of praise for the Indians and their canoes. "I must give these Savages as well as those on the coast the praise of making the neatest handsomest lightest best formed canoes I ever saw & are the best hands to work them."

The route up the Columbia led through country heavily populated, and the Corps met Indians all along the shore. Some had fish but were not in a mood to sell. They preferred to sell dogs. The word had obviously gone around that dogs were a saleable item. The Indians wanted tobacco in exchange for the dogs, but there was none to spare. Most of the men were confirmed smokers, and when they ran out of tobacco they chewed or smoked a bitter bark they had found to be a good substitute. The Indians were as fond of tobacco as the men of the Corps, although the Indian tobacco was not the same as the Virginian leaves the men had brought with them. Eventually there was no more, and the smokers could not wait until they reached the caches on the other side of the mountains where they had stored tobacco.

Deer became easier to hunt, although many of them were skinny and not much use for food. On the many islands along the south shore were huge flocks of waterfowl, sandhill cranes, and swans. The migration season up the West Coast flyway was in full swing. The winter birds were preparing to go north, and the summer birds were already coming in.

Wildlife grew abundant. On April 5, Lewis recorded seeing a tick. Although it looked somewhat the same as the ones Lewis had been used to in the East, it was probably an *Ixodes pacificus,* the western black-legged tick, a carrier of Lyme disease. Ticks lie in wait on grass and bushes, and when a furred animal or a person wearing clothes brushes against them, they have no difficulty in attaching themselves to the passer-by, then finding a suitable spot, typically on the neck or groin—these areas of the body offer warmth and epidermal blood vessels—to eat a meal of blood. Their attachment to the skin is assisted by a biological cement that makes removal difficult. The larvae of some ticks are no bigger than a printed period (.) and are almost impossible to see until they become engorged with blood. No one likes to walk around with a bloated tick on his or her neck. If a tick is a disease carrier, the longer it remains attached and the more it becomes bloated with blood, the greater the chance of its host being infected. Just as the men spent time trying to rid themselves of fleas while at Fort Clatsop, they may well have sat around the fire searching each other for ticks, although there was then no known connection between ticks and disease.

As the expedition proceeded up the river they were constantly meeting Indians who, out of curiosity, invited them to visit their villages. Lewis learned of some strange customs. One tribe bathed their bodies with urine every morning, but also made frequent use of sweat baths. The burial of the dead was a constant source of interest. Most of the Indians along the river wrapped their dead in cloth and laid them in a canoe that was placed on a special island for the dead. The canoe, elaborately carved and decorated and filled with items of travel to the spirit world, was raised on ornamental

---

I stood near the Columbia River, binoculars to my eyes, watching some sparrows on a nearby bush. It was April 5, 1995. Suddenly a hummingbird flew across my line of vision. It came and went with such speed that I could not identify it except as a hummingbird. But that evening, rereading Lewis' journal, I came across this entry. "Saturday April 5th 1806 . . . saw the log cock, the humming bird, Geese, Duck to-day. The tick has made its appearance it is the same with those of the Atlantic States." Nature's clock had not changed, and the hummingbirds still arrive on time. The log cock was the pileated woodpecker, a handsome, large black woodpecker with a prominent red crest on its head.

---

wooden pylons, with the feet of the corpse facing downstream. Other groups disposed of the dead by laying them in what Lewis called a vault, a roofed platform above ground, on which the corpses might be laid, three or four thick, one upon the other.

While the tribes along the river were not as nomadic as the Plains Indians, they followed the salmon harvest. When the fish were running in the spring and summer they moved to where they could catch and dry fish, then moved back to winter quarters after the run of fish had finished. So it was not unusual to find a village with empty houses from which the people had temporarily moved away.

As the men moved slowly back up the river they were told of a river the Indians called the Multnomah (now the Willamette), which they had missed on the way down. Clark backtracked and explored the river until he was told about falls higher up that would block his way. While investigating one camp he found the locals "sulkey" and reluctant to sell him food. So to induce them to sell he played a dirty little magic trick on them, dropping some "portfire"—a piece of string impregnated with gunpowder and used to start a campfire—into the cooking fire in the middle of their hut. There was an immediate flash of blue flame. At the same time, like a magician showing off his tricks, he spun the needle on a compass with the aid of a magnet. The old ladies were scared and implored him to stop, and the village shaman began to appeal loudly to his gods. When the fire died down the people were only too happy to give Clark food, without asking a price for it. Clark did eventually pay for the food, but the practical joke cannot have endeared him to the locals. "I lit my pipe and gave them smoke & gave the womin the full price of the roots they had put at my feet. They appeared Somewhat passified and I left them and proceeded on. . . ."

The attitudes of Lewis and Clark toward both the Indians and the men were changing. For whatever reason, their tempers flared in ways that had not happened on the outward journey. Perhaps the change was due to the stress of facing the hazards of the return trip; perhaps it was the length of their separation from home while constantly being surrounded by danger; perhaps it was the never-ending closeness of living with all the others. Lewis was more volatile than Clark, and on many occasions there was a good excuse for him to lose his temper. The Indians along the river were a slippery-fingered lot and did not hesitate to steal any small item that the men left lying unguarded around the camp. Even Seaman, Lewis' dog, was stolen. Lewis' reaction was swift and furious. He sent out a recovery party with instructions to shoot if the dog was not returned. The Indians quickly gave up the dog. This was the first time Lewis gave specific instructions to shoot, even without a direct threat to the lives of the men.

On several occasions Lewis blazed with anger and told the local people that if they continued to steal they would be punished. Despite the fact that he did not speak a word of their language, his yelling and screaming and thrashing the air with a stick must have made it abundantly clear what he thought and what he was going to do. Lewis became convinced that it was only the size and strength of the party that was preventing them from being attacked and killed. The guards were instructed to be especially vigilant, and no baggage was allowed to lie unattended. No one had raised a hand against an Indian on the outward journey, but more than once during the return journey, Lewis flogged an Indian for stealing. Flogging was an accepted punishment in the U.S. military, and Lewis' reaction reflected his military training and authority. In one place the Chief was very apologetic and complained that the trouble was due to a couple of hot-blooded young men. The men of the Corps were young and equally hot-blooded and would not have hesitated to fight, had the orders been given. Discretion became the better part of anger. Tempers flared but died down. No shots were fired and no one was killed.

Later, when the Corps was with the Nez Percé Indians, Lewis became involved in a shouting match with a young man who taunted him for eating dog and threw a puppy into his dinner. Lewis caught the puppy and threw it back at the Indian, striking him in the face. At the same time he seized his tomahawk, leaped to his feet, and threatened the Indian with violence if he continued in his "impertinence." The Indian retreated, shamefaced.

It goes without saying that not all the Indians were dishonest or thieves. On one rapid, when a canoe was being hauled up over the rocks, the towrope broke and the canoe floated back down. The Indians at the foot of the rapid recovered the canoe and hauled it back up again to return it. They could have easily kept it. Later in the journey other Indians returned items that had been lost and were praised in the journals for their honesty.

As the Corps progressed toward the mountains the Indians gave them alarming news. The expected run of salmon had not materialized, and the people higher up the river were starving. This was a matter of grave concern, not only for the Indians but for the Corps who expected to live off fresh salmon until they got back to an area where there would either be horses or game to eat. The hunters were sent out in every direction and, with good luck, brought back enough meat to tide them over a period of hardship. It was dried over open fires in the forest and stored in bags of elk hide. Poor, starving Indians scrabbled around the edge of the camp picking up scraps of meat and bone the men left behind.

The current in the river became stronger as the Corps moved closer to the rapids, through which they had exultantly run their boats on the way down, against the advice of the Indians who had stood on the bank expecting to witness a drowning. Now they had a hard portage, emptying the canoes and hauling them upstream by elk skin ropes. Some relief was available. They had arrived again at the land of the horse and, for a price, were able to buy some horses to help carry the loads. The horses were expensive—two cooking kettles for four horses, reducing the messes to one small kettle each in which to prepare their food. The horses they bought were stallions because the local people, not as used to horses as other tribes, did not know the art of gelding. It was the breeding season and the horses were wild and difficult to restrain, even though they were hobbled and tied to pickets.

The same day they bought horses the Indians caught the first salmon—an occasion for great rejoicing. The first fish was cooked and divided into small pieces and given to the children of the village. The Indians promised that a big run of fish would start within five days. This time, they proved to be wrong. The fish did not arrive until the Corps was ready to cross the mountains, and they never reaped the benefit of unlimited salmon.

By April 20, 1806, there had been only one mention in the journals about the men who were sick when they left Fort Clatsop. On April 11, Lewis, faced with the problem of portaging a rapid, had written: "This portage is two thousand eight hundred yards along a rough narrow and slipery road. The duty of getting the canoes above the rapid was by mutual consent confided to my friend Capt. C. who took with him for that purpose all the party except Bratton who is yet so weak he is unable to walk, three others who were lamed by various accidents and one other to cook for the party." On April 20, Bratton was still *hors de combat* and "compelled to ride as he was yet unable to walk." What had happened to him in the previous month? If his back made it impossible to walk, he was presumably unable to paddle. There had been mention of buying dogs to supplement the diet for the sick men, but no word of treatment or the severity of Bratton's disability. This is hard to explain, considering that just before the departure from Fort Clatsop Lewis had been concerned that Bratton might not recover.

The expedition was now entering the country of the Walla-Walla, a friendly tribe with a culture based on horses. The land flattened into a plain and there would be no further need for the canoes. Horses would be better. In an act of spite that in retrospect seems petty, the canoes were burned so that none of the Indians they had found so annoying could make use of them. The men loaded their packhorses and started leading them toward the distant mountains that were still covered with snow.

Minor troubles still annoyed Lewis. He continued to be suspicious of the Indians, whom he called "pore, durty and haughty." Charbonneau's horse threw its load and went charging off with a robe flapping from the saddle, frightening the horse even more. When the horse was caught the robe had already been stolen and hidden in one of the Indian's lodges. Lewis was so angry that he threatened to burn down the Indian's house if the robe was not returned. This extraordinary threat was the culmination of repeated acts of thievery that were driving Lewis to the brink of potentially disastrous retaliation. He was probably equally miffed because his *bête noir,* Charbonneau, had been responsible for the horse. The following day Charbonneau blundered again because more horses for which he was responsible broke their tethers and strayed. The same thing happened a few days later, and poor Charbonneau was again the named culprit. These frustrations always took place in the morning and delayed the departure of the train of packhorses. Lewis' temper was not improving.

The route from the Columbia River to the Rocky Mountains lay across a stony plain where walking was hard. The men had not been marching for a long time, and many of them, including Lewis, complained of sore feet. "My left ankle gives me much pain. I baithed my feet in cold water from which I experienced considerable relief."

The Corps proceeded on, accompanied by a retinue of Indians. Some of the hazards they had met earlier reappeared. They killed several rattlesnakes, but no one was bitten. One evening Cruzatte brought out his fiddle at the request of the natives and the men danced. A good sign. Cruzatte, the merrymaker, had not played for a long time.

Food was running short, but Lady Luck played into their hands yet again. A very friendly Wallawallah Chief, Yellept, appeared and invited them to come to his camp where he would be able to supply them with both horses and food. Yellept made a speech to his people and urged them to help the expedition. He set an example himself by bringing the Corps firewood and three roasted mullet. Lewis bought four dogs and they "suped heartily having been on short allowance for two days." The next morning Yellept presented Clark with "a very elegant white horse." He wanted a kettle in return, but when told that they had no more kettles they could afford to lose, he was happy with whatever they gave to him. A pleasant difference from the contentious haggling that had been the rule for several weeks.

During the next few days several Indians displayed their honesty. One man walked 26 miles to catch up with the group and return some steel traps that had been left behind at his village.

Another returned a horse that had escaped. Both these kind deeds were rewarded with gifts, and the Captains recorded them in their journals with pleasure.

Eight months before, on the journey west, the horses the expedition had acquired were left in the care of Twisted Hair, one of many Nez Percé Chiefs. When he appeared in camp he immediately got into a shouting match with another Chief, Cut Nose. Lewis could not understand what the argument was about. The language had to pass through six different interpretations to be understood. Eventually, however, it came out that Twisted Hair had been careless about the handling of the expedition's horses and saddles, a lack of responsibility to which Cut Nose objected. Around an evening campfire the dispute was settled, and during the next few days most of the horses were found and returned.

The medical skills of both Captains, and particularly Clark, were called into play intensively during the next weeks. Progress through the mountains was delayed by deep snow, and the expedition had to spend about five weeks with the Nez Percé waiting impatiently for the spring thaw to open the trails. They did not realize that, in the Rockies, deep snow frequently persists well into June and even into July, and the winter that was ending had been one with very heavy snowfall. The expedition could either try to push ahead prematurely, against the advice of the natives, and get into trouble, or bide their time until the route became passable. During the wait Clark's medical skills proved both useful and profitable.

The list of the sick and injured Indians was long and interesting. One man had a knee contracted by "rheumatism," several had broken arms, and a multitude of people came with eye problems. Ordway wrote: "Our officers dressed their wounds, washed their eyes & gave them meddicine and told them how to apply it &c." The scene, which was to be repeated many times during the next few weeks, was almost biblical. The poor, the halt, and the lame came to be healed by an almost mystical foreigner whose medicine seemed more magical than their own. Even the songs the men sang around the campfire were regarded as "medicine songs" by the Indians, who wanted to learn them and gain their power.

Eye problems had been common with the men of the expedition and were very prevalent among the Nez Percé. Lewis thought they were due to fine sand blown into the eyes by the ever-present wind. Some complaints may have been due to this, but it is far more likely that most were caused by infectious conjunctivitis ("pink eye"), trachoma, or gonorrhea. Conjunctivitis is a bacterial infection of the lining of the eyelids. It is easily acquired and as easily spread. A child rubs his gummed-up, swollen, and irritated eye and then scratches and infects his other eye. An attentive mother wipes both eyes with the tail of a garment and, without washing her own hands, rubs her own eyes. She becomes infected and the infection passes down the chain. Similar lack of hygiene causes the spread of gonorrheal conjunctivitis, a more serious form of the disease that can lead to blindness and ulcers on the cornea. As venereal diseases were common in all the Indian tribes, many people, both men, women, and children must have been infected with gonorrheal conjunctivitis, and children born through an infected birth canal easily acquire the neonatal form of the disease. Nowadays, gonorrheal eye infections are readily cured with antibiotics. If they are not quickly cured they become chronic and the cause of constant distress and, possibly, blindness.

Trachoma, at one time called Egyptian ophthalmia because of its widespread occurrence in the Middle East, is a miserable, painful, and uncomfortable chronic inflammation of the conjunctiva caused by *Chlamydia trachomatis*. The infection starts innocently enough with a little swelling and irritation of the eye but progresses to scarring of the conjunctiva, and the eyelashes turn inward and constantly scratch the cornea, which also becomes scarred and ulcerated. The end-point is a blind, scarred eye, now curable in its early stages, but back then, incurable.

The medicine most commonly dispensed by Clark—for he soon became the doctor of choice for the Indians—was "eye water," a mixture of zinc sulfate (white vitriol) and lead acetate (sugar of lead). Benjamin Rush had a prescription for making up two quarts of the mixture in snowmelt or springwater, and he advised that the eyes be bathed with the mixture three or four times a day. Most of the Indians probably had their eyes washed only once, although a vial of eye water was given to one Chief to distribute to his people.

The sick lined up in droves. One morning Clark had more than forty patients waiting for his attention. There were perhaps more eye problems than others, but men also came with badly set broken bones, and women complained of weakness in the loins. Diagnosis of some of the conditions would be difficult even now, and must have been a complete mystery to Clark, but he did not seem to fear making a mistake. He was sheltered by the simple theories of disease of the time, and if he really believed Benjamin Rush's ideas, everyone suffered from some form of a single disease. If he had known what a modern doctor knows he would have been frustrated by his inability to make a precise diagnosis or provide treatment with the limited resources at his command.

The situations Clark faced are still pertinent today. Practicing medicine as a doctor traveling in a third-world country, trekking in

---

Zinc sulfate was a common component of eye medicines in the nineteenth century. Zinc has some antibiotic properties and, used as a solution and eye wash, helped to reduce infection. Ophthalmic textbooks of that era advised that the eyes be bathed several times a day. One text said, "Eye-waters and drops are solutions of astringent, stimulant or narcotic substances, or of all combined. . . . Eye-waters properly so called, are the weaker solutions, and are used to bathe the eye occasionally in the course of the day." Lead acetate, the other component of Clark's eye water was later found to be harmful to the eye, sometimes precipitating as an opacity on the cornea. Eyedrops containing antibiotics and steroids have long since supplanted zinc and lead acetate for the cure of eye infections.

Nepal, exploring jungles in Borneo, or climbing in Peru on an "adventure" trip, pose similar ethical questions as those faced by Clark. Imagine a poor, dirty, sick, but heartbreakingly charming old woman hobbling up, asking for help. The nearest doctor is 100 miles away, the nearest hospital 500 miles away. The patient has never been outside her village and has no money to travel or see a doctor. The visiting doctor cannot understand what the patient is saying, and local customs forbid an examination of anything but the patient's hands and face. The diagnosis becomes a wild guess, based on limited knowledge of local diseases, prevalent parasites, and the statistical possibilities. Treatment depends on what is available in the doctor's pack—an antibiotic, an antimalarial pill, or an aspirin. The doctor has no idea of the woman's past history and possible allergies to medication. Good instructions about how and when to take the medicine cannot be given, and it is impossible to leave enough pills for a full course of treatment. The doctor may be fairly sure that the woman has tuberculosis, so, like Clark trying to do no harm, gives her a couple of aspirin, pats her on the back, and moves on, his conscience hurting.

During the past few years ethical questions have been raised about treating unknown patients in an isolated situation. Lewis asked the same questions. On the outgoing journey Clark treated an old man with a painful knee. His treatment was simple and appropriate: liniment. The man recovered and never ceased to sing the praises of the white doctor and his medicine. There is nothing more helpful to a doctor's practice than a grateful patient. "My friend Capt. C. is their favorite phisician and has already received many applications," wrote Lewis who was astute enough to realize that the confidence of the people in eye water not only added to the benefit of the treatment but gave the patients an inflated view of Clark's skill. This presented an ethical dilemma. Should the Indians be told that Clark was not a doctor, or should he continue to treat the people without disclosing the truth?

The Indians would not have known the difference between a trained doctor and a charlatan. To them, Clark was a kind, attentive medicine man who was able to cure their painful eyes. To Lewis, the problem was more complicated. They had been receiving important and sometimes valuable gifts in return for minor medical attention. Clark received a "very eligant grey mare" in exchange for a bottle of eye water. The horse could carry Clark across the mountains; the eye water would provide relief for a day or two. Lewis made his decision. "In our present situation I think it is pardonable to continue this deseption for they will not give us any provision without compensation in merchandise and our stock is now reduced to a mere handful. We take care to give them no article which can possibly injure them." One of the oldest principles in medicine is "Do no harm." Both Lewis and Clark were fulfilling the principle in a compassionate way and within the limits of their knowledge. Some of their treatments could have done harm, but their medical background, based on the theories of the age, could not let them know that. For obvious, practical, and benevolent reasons, they continued to treat the Indians.

For nearly a month Lewis wrote nothing about the health of his own men. Then, on May 24, Bratton's case came up again. "William Bratton still continues very unwell. He eats heartily digests his food well and has recovered his flesh almost perfectly is so weak in the loins that he is scarcely able to walk, nor can he set upwright but with the greatest pain. We have tried every remidy which our enginuity could devise, or which our stock of medicines furnish us, without effect." What followed was dramatic and hard to explain.

John Shields told Lewis that he had heard that sweat baths sometimes cured people with conditions similar to Bratton's. Nothing ventured, nothing gained. Bratton, no doubt desperate for a cure, agreed to the sweat bath. A pit was dug, 3 feet across by 4 feet deep, with a fire on its floor. When the fire had heated the bottom and sides of the hole, the embers were removed and a wooden seat and footrest placed within it. Bratton, naked, was lowered into the hole that was then covered by a roof of willow wands and blankets. Water was poured on the heated soil so that he sat in a steam-filled oven. He was given two twenty-minute treatments, with a plunge into cold water in between. Finally he sat in the hole for forty-five minutes, drinking copious drafts of mint tea. He was removed, wrapped in blankets, and allowed to cool slowly. Within twenty-four hours he was up, walking, and almost free of pain.

What had been wrong with Bratton? He was first reported to be sick on February 10 and was miraculously cured by a single sweat on May 23. (Lewis wrote about the sweat bath on May 24.) Earlier in Bratton's illness the symptoms were typical of a slipped inter-vertebral disc: onset of pain during heavy work at the salt camp, back pain radiating into the thigh and leg, inability to work or walk, but with generally good maintenance of his weight and "flesh." The pattern fit the diagnosis except for the episode of fever that accom-panied the first pain. He could have had flu at the same time as a slipped disc, but doctors like to join different symptoms in a single diagnosis, and this is sometimes difficult to do. Herniated—slipped—discs do occasionally pop back into position spontaneously, and, if the disc problem was associated with muscle spasms, the heat of the sweat bath could have relieved the spasms and helped the disc return to its normal position.

The primary problem, whatever the diagnosis, was in Bratton's lower back, within the spinal canal, or adjacent to the vertebral col-umn, thus irritating nerves going to the legs. Neither a malignant nor a benign tumor could have been cured in a sauna. An infection of one of the vertebral bones has been suggested, but, once again, such a quick cure seems an unlikely outcome for a bone infection. An acute infection would have caused the fever, but the fever did not continue as might have been expected with a persistent prob-lem. A serious infection such as tuberculosis would have caused progressive deterioration in Bratton's condition. He would have lost weight and become a pale, thin shadow of his former vigorous self. He did not. He remained in good health except for the pain in his back and legs.

Many conditions cause lower back pain, but there are few prob-lems that would go away spontaneously. After consulting with several orthopedic and neurosurgeons, the best conclusion is that

Bratton had a herniated disc with muscle spasms. The heat relieved the spasms and the disc relocated spontaneously.

The story of a paralyzed Indian Chief was, if anything, more mysterious than that of Bratton. The Indians brought Clark a well-known Chief, a man of "considerable estate," who had been a quadriplegic for at least three years. (One note says five years, another says three.) He had never been injured, and Lewis quickly noticed that, in spite of his paralysis, the Chief had not lost weight and his limbs looked normal. He had been unable to move his limbs and had lain like a corpse in whatever position he was placed, but he ate heartily, was normal intellectually, and had a strong pulse. Apart from being pale from lack of exposure, he looked like a normal man. Lewis thought that the diet of roots eaten by the Indians caused this illness and all the disorders of the natives, except rheumatism. The Chief was urged to change his diet to fish and meat and to take a cold bath every morning. He was given cream of tartar, a laxative and diuretic, and flowers of sulfur, a laxative that would also induce sweating, to take every three days.

The Chief was brought to camp for a second visit, about the time that Bratton was cured, but his condition had not changed: no pain, and still unable to use his limbs. Lewis wrote, "nor do we suppose that it can be a paralytic attack or his limbs should have been diminished." Lewis was basing his opinion on what he must have seen in other paralyzed people with thin, wasted limbs: an astute and knowledgeable observation. There was no improvement although "the poor wretch" thought he was a little better. He was given some laudanum and portable soup.

In light of Bratton's rapid recovery, and in response to an appeal by the patient himself, Lewis ordered the sweat bath that had been used with Bratton to be heated up again. There was an unforeseen problem. The paralyzed Chief could not be lowered into the pit that was only 3 feet across. Lewis was, nevertheless, determined to proceed with the treatment and informed the Indian's companions that the only hope of a cure would be "sefere swetts."

Two days later another attempt was made. The hole was enlarged and the sick man, supported by his father who had been very attentive, was lowered into it. The sweat was not satisfactory, and the Chief suffered from pain so severe that he required laudanum for relief. One day later the Chief was much improved and could use his hands and arms and "was much pleased with the prospect of recovery." He felt better than he had in months. The care bestowed by the family on the sick man impressed Lewis, who thought that the Nez Percé were kinder to their old and their women than the other tribes they had met.

Both Bratton and the Chief continued to improve. Within two days of his second sweat the Chief was able to wash his face himself, something he had not been able to do for a year. He was quickly given another sweat, after which he could move his legs and toes, and his arms were completely better. Naturally, he was delighted and Lewis was hopeful of a complete recovery. Lewis thought that the Chief would have been an ideal patient for electricity, a therapy he knew was being used in Philadelphia.

Hazarding a guess about the Chief's diagnosis is even more difficult than in Bratton's case. The critical evidence was that he had not lost any musculature, despite years of paralysis. His body looked as good as that of a healthy man. Lewis did not see or recognize mental illness in the Indians, except in a few isolated cases. Was the Chief hysterical? Was he a malingerer? Perhaps he enjoyed the attention he received from his family and the relief from the arduous duties of hunting and fighting that his illness brought him. An organic disease of the nervous system, such as poliomyelitis, would have left him with wasted limbs that could never have responded to heat treatment. Were the cures of Bratton and the Chief connected psychologically? The Chief's family asked for a sweat because of its success with Bratton. Regardless of the diagnosis the treatment was successful, and the Chief's recovery can only have enhanced the medical reputation of the Captains and their "miraculous" treatments.

Taking care of the sick continued to keep "Dr." Clark busy. While Bratton and the Chief were being treated, little Baptiste, now fifteen months old, and of whom Clark was fond, became very sick on May 22. "Charbono's child is very ill this evening; he is cutting teeth, and for several days past has had a violent lax, which having suddenly stopped he was attacked with a high fever and his neck and throat are much swolen this evening." He, like Bratton and the Chief, was treated with cream of tartar and flowers of sulfur, and a poultice of boiled wild onions was applied to his neck, as hot as the child could tolerate it. The clear intent was to draw the infection to a "head."

A day later the medications had worked on Baptiste's bowels, but the developing abscess had abated little. The poultice was applied several times a day, but the abscess became worse with even more swelling, although there was some decrease in his fever. Baptiste's fever must have been assessed by the time-honored laying of a hand on the forehead and, perhaps, by judging how much he was sweating. The only thermometer, used for measuring the temperature of air and water, had been broken weeks before.

By May 25, three days after the start of his illness, Baptiste was worse and a source of great worry to the camp. Clark administered more cream of tartar and flowers of sulfur, which did not work, so the boy was given an enema, which worked. Twenty-four hours later Lewis wrote, "The Clyster given to the child last evening operated very well. It is clear of fever this evening and is much better, the swelling is considerably abated and appears as if it would pass off without coming to a head. We still continue the fresh poltices of onions to the swollen part." Within a day Baptiste was better, although Lewis believed the swelling would still develop into a boil ("imposthume") just below the left ear. The infection continued on its anticipated course. Baptiste's fever broke, and the boil seemed to be advancing to "maturity" and was getting ready to burst. He clearly had a pharyngeal abscess or an infected lymph gland in the neck, and it was fortunate that it healed without bursting. The poultice helped the inflammation to localize. There was no special benefit from the onions; probably any hot, wet poultice would have had the same effect.

As the sick improved, Lewis had other worries on his mind. There were no more trade goods, and the men were reduced to cutting the brass buttons off their uniforms to exchange for food. They had no desire to repeat the privations of the previous fall and wanted to prepare for the journey over the Rocky Mountains, "where hunger and cold in their most rigorous assail the wearied traveler; not any of us has forgotten our sufferings in those mountains in September last, and I think it probable we never shall." Their trading efforts were successful and they collected three bushels of roots. Two tomahawks that had been stolen were also retrieved, one a touching memento.

One of the tomahawks had belonged to Sergeant Floyd and had been carefully carried halfway across the continent and back, to be returned to the Sergeant's family. The old man found with the tomahawk had bought it from the thief, and he himself was about to die. His relatives were reluctant to give up the tomahawk because they intended to bury it with the old man when he died. The trade was expensive; two strands of beads and two horses that would be killed at the grave of the man after he had died. Honor was served on both sides. The Sergeant's tomahawk would be returned to his family, and the old man would have two horses to ride into the spirit world. The tomahawk, with its sentimental value, had never been mentioned before, and was never mentioned again.

By June 3, Bratton was walking without pain or disability, and the Chief was recovering the use of all his limbs. Baptiste was better, and his boil had resolved into a hard lump below the ear. The poultices continued, and over the next few days the inflammation subsided completely. In the meantime, the efforts to obtain food proved rewarding. Ordway, Frazier, and Weiser returned from a 70-mile shopping trip with seventeen salmon. It was a long way to the marketplace, and because of the length of the journey, some of the salmon were inedible.

The urge to get going across the mountains was strong. The Indians told Lewis that perhaps they could cross the mountains in a couple of weeks, when more snow had melted. In the meantime, they had sent a messenger across the mountains to find out the state of affairs and bring news of what had happened during the winter. Lewis thought that if an Indian could cross the mountains, so could his men.

The Indians had promised guides to lead the Corps through the mountains, but seemed to be dillydallying in selecting them. The food supply, however, was improving, and Lewis concluded that, as a result of successful trading, they had enough bread and roots for the next stage of their voyage. They had collected sixty-five horses so that each man could ride and also have a packhorse. The final days were spent preparing saddles, filled with goat hair, and packing their loads.

A final entry about the Chief, dated June 8, 1806, confirmed his continued progress. He could stand and had regained much of his strength, perhaps because he had never lost the mass of his muscles. Bratton was no longer considered an invalid. Lewis remarked, "He has had a tedious illness which he boar with much fortitude and firmness."

Lewis wanted his men, who had not been marching for several weeks, to exercise and train themselves for the tough trip ahead. It seems surprising that men who could make a 70-mile trek to buy only seventeen fish would need much reconditioning. But they ran foot races against the Indians and played "prison base," a children's game that involved a lot of running. Indian Chiefs dropped by the camp to say farewell and trade for the last horses. The river, beside which they had been camping, was falling, an indication that the snowmelt was finishing. Just a few more days waiting would dry the trails and improve the grass for the horses.

On June 10, 1806, the Corps of Discovery left on the next momentous stage of their journey, feeling themselves "perfectly equiped for the mountains." Each man had his own horse and a packhorse to carry a light load. Extra horses were taken in case of accidents and as a supply of food. Optimism must have been high. They had been waiting several weeks for the snow to melt, and now they were moving again.

The Weippe Prairies afforded a good camping ground for a few days' rest and hunting. The hunters brought in eight deer, and turkey vultures ate another before it could be retrieved. Rain was falling on the morning of June 15, so they delayed their departure for an hour but left when it was obvious the rain would not let up. The rain had made the trail slippery, and several of the horses fell. Progress was slow and difficult. They had to cross a creek three times, and fallen timber made the march hazardous for the horses. Lewis was as observant as ever and found the nest of a hummingbird with eggs: a tiny cup of grass, balanced precariously on the top of a branch. In spite of difficulties the Corps went 22 miles that day.

The following morning they made an early start, rode a number of miles, then stopped to allow the horses to feed. Patches of deep snow in shady places were an ominous sign. Hints of spring were hard to find, an occasional flower and a few new leaves. Columbine, flowering pea, and angelica graced the spots where the snow had melted. The farther they went, the deeper the snow became. Fortunately, it was firm enough to hold the horses, but in places was still 8 to 10 feet deep. They went 15 miles and camped at Hungry Creek.

The next morning brought a halt to their attempt to cross the mountains. The snow was 12 to 15 feet deep, even on the sunny side of the slopes. The air was cold and Lewis' hands and feet were "benumbed." There was no hope they could reach the next place where there would be food for the horses, and even the indefatigable Drewyer was not sure he could find the way along the ridges. If they proceeded, everything could be lost: horses, men, instruments, and journals. Disappointed, they turned back. The first defeat of the expedition. They resolved to cache much of their baggage where they had stopped, turn back, camp at a suitable place with feed for the horses, find an Indian guide, and try again in a few days. They returned to a place near Hungry Creek, and, as though to depress their spirits even more, rain fell all evening.

Drewyer and Shannon were sent ahead to find Indian guides, offering rifles as payment for services. While they were away, Potts cut his leg badly with a large knife and bled profusely from a big vein on the inner side of his leg. Lewis had trouble stopping the bleeding until he wrapped a tight bandage over a small piece of wood to apply pressure to the bleeding point. To add to the problems, Colter's horse fell and both tumbled down into a creek. Luckily, neither Colter nor the horse was injured. A pleasant campsite was found and the hunters were sent out. They killed no deer, but food for the horses was abundant.

Lewis' major worry was that if they could not make their way through the mountains soon, they would never reach the United States before another winter. He was determined to try again quickly by sending a strong, small advance party ahead to find and prepare the route.

Some Indians came to the camp and said that Drewyer and Shannon, who had been sent to find guides, would not be back for a couple of days. The reason for this was not clear. So, delayed in this way, the hunters went out and killed eight deer and three bears. The salmon were running, at long last, and the expedition was able to stock up on food. Potts' leg was in pain, and Lewis applied a poultice of camas roots to the inflamed part.

Drewyer and Shannon returned with three Indians who had agreed to guide the Corps to the Great Falls of the Missouri. The guides were all known to be reliable men and "much respected by their nation." On June 24, the expedition started back up into the mountains, after the Indians had set trees ablaze to bring good luck.

Travel conditions were better. Snow that had been 10 feet deep was now 7 feet deep and firm enough to support the horses. This made progress easier. The snow covered many of the fallen trees and rocks that would have made progress difficult for the horses. Their cached supplies were still intact. The Indian guides wanted to push ahead to a place where the horses could feed.

The route continued along the ridges, and at the highest point, the group stopped to smoke a pipe where generations of Indians had built a mound of stones 8 feet high, crowned by a tall pine pole. Building cairns at the summits of passes and ridges is a common response to the rigors of a climb. In the Himalayas the cairns are topped by strings of prayer flags flapping in the wind. Each passing pilgrim adds another stone or another flag. A modern climber or Sherpa would have immediately understood the significance of the cairns.

The route was still dangerous. Lewis' horse slipped while descending the side of a creek, and Lewis fell 40 feet before he could stop himself. The horse nearly fell on top of him, but both escaped unharmed. After six days of travel—much easier than the eleven days of torment on the way west—the expedition reached Traveler's Rest.

At this point Lewis and Clark acted upon a plan they had made while camped at Fort Clatsop. Lewis wanted to explore the Marias River to find out where it originated and how far north it went. On the way west they had been told that there were easier routes through the mountains. The plan was to split the group so that both the Marias and the Yellowstone rivers could be explored. Lewis would take the most direct route to the Great Falls. There, some of his party would accompany him up the Marias and then return to the Missouri, while the remainder of his group portaged around the falls. Clark would take an entirely different route. He would lead a party to the Three Forks of the Missouri, at which point they would also split into two smaller parties: one to go down the Yellowstone and the other to go overland by horse to the Mandan villages. All being well, the whole group, Lewis, and Clark, would rendezvous at the mouth of the Yellowstone.

It was understandable that Lewis would want to explore the Marias and determine how far north the American territory extended, but a military tactician would have questioned his judgment. The expedition was reentering the plains where the threat from aggressive Indians would be greatest, a time when they should have been at maximum strength. Instead, they were splitting up into several small, vulnerable groups, one of which was going to go by land on horses across a landscape where the Indians were the masters. The Nez Percé guides had warned them they might be killed. The land may have appeared empty, but there were bands of hunting and fighting Indians everywhere. It was a dangerous place.

Lewis called for volunteers to go with him. He chose Drewyer, the Fields brothers, William Werner, Frazier and Sergeant Gass. All the others would go with Clark. On July 3, the parties went their separate ways. Lewis wrote, "We saddled our horses and set out I took leave of my worthy friend and companion Capt. Clark. . . . I could not avoid feeling much concern on this occasion although I hoped the separation was only momentary." This was one of the most touching moments in the whole voyage. The two men had become inseparable companions, trusting each other, relying on the other's judgment and strength. And now they would part, not knowing if they would ever meet again.

The Indian guides who had started out with Lewis soon left to go another way. They were afraid of meeting the Minnetare Indians. Lewis so appreciated their guiding the Corps through the mountains that he gave them a generous supply of meat. The farewell to "these affectionate people" was touched with genuine sadness.

There were signs of Minnetare war parties all along the trail and Lewis noted, without seeming alarmed, that, "they have a large pasel of horses." His party expected to meet a war party and were on their guard day and night, but no matter what the danger, Lewis continued to fill his journal with descriptions of flowers and animals. He also noted that the mosquitoes were so ferocious they had to build smoky fires to protect the horses. The hunters had no difficulty in shooting deer for the pot, and Drewyer killed two beaver, one of which bit him badly on the knee. Wolves, goats, and elk were becoming more common, and Joseph Fields killed the first buffalo they had seen for many months. Within two days Lewis was again seeing thousands of buffalo. Meat would no longer be in short supply, but the horses, coming from the western side of the mountains, had never seen buffalo before and were greatly alarmed by their bellowing.

Lewis' groups met the Missouri at the White Bear Island and shot eleven buffalo for meat and for hides to make canoes to cross the river. After they had crossed over to the southern side of the river they opened the cache that had been buried so many months before. The bearskins, the plant specimens, and the medicines had deteriorated. The chart of the Missouri was still intact. The old carriage wheels were dug up, and the iron frame of the collapsible boat was also still in good order.

Meanwhile, Drewyer, who had been sent to look for horses that had probably been stolen by Indians, had not rejoined the men, greatly worrying Lewis. To Lewis' relief, Drewyer returned after two days, but without the horses. He had followed the trail of the horses and found a deserted Indian camp with fifteen lodges. The Indians, probably on a buffalo hunt, had stolen the horses, and there was no hope of getting them back. Lewis had been concerned that Drewyer might have been attacked by a bear, knowing that if he became separated from his horse he would almost certainly be killed. "I felt so perfectly satisfied that he had returned to safety that I thought but little of the horses although they were seven of the best I had." They still had ten horses, including the two best and the two worst.

Alarms and worries were constant companions. One morning all the horses had disappeared but were soon found again. Grizzlies roamed throughout the area, making it dangerous to search for firewood, but they were nothing compared with the possibility of meeting a war party of Indians up the Marias. All the men were worried about meeting with Minnetares or Blackfeet Indians. "They are a vicious lawless and rather abandoned set of wretches I wish to avoid an interview with them if possible." Lewis knew that if only their horses and supplies were stolen, at best it would be a long walk home. At worst, it would be the end of them.

Lewis headed north up the Marias on July 17. He took with him Drewyer and the two Fields brothers. They were the best hunters and, therefore, probably the best marksmen. If he could not take a large party, at least he could take the best. Werner, Frazier, and Sergeant Gass were left to portage the falls. Almost immediately Lewis found a bleeding buffalo and thought it had been wounded recently by Indians. Lewis climbed a small hill and scanned the plains with his telescope. He saw nothing alarming. During the next few days his party slowly ascended the Marias River, killing buffalo for meat. At night they kept watch, Lewis taking his turn with the men. As they went north the plains became more desolate, the soil thinner, and the buffalo fewer. The gravel hurt the horses feet, which made travel slower. Eventually they discerned that the river would not lead them where they had hoped and decided to rest for a couple of days and take astronomical observations. There were signs of Indians everywhere.

The observations were obscured by bad weather and clouds, and Lewis called the northernmost camp, Camp Disappointment. On the afternoon of July 26, Lewis had barely left camp before he saw a group of about thirty horses and some Indians silhouetted on a ridge about a mile away. The scene was ominous. It was the very one they had wanted to avoid. Half the horses were saddled, and Lewis, using his spyglass, soon realized that the Indians were not looking at him, but down into the valley where Drewyer was hunting. "This was a very unpleasant sight. However I resolved to approach them and make the best of our situation."

The next hours were filled with tension and drama. When the Indians discovered Lewis and the Fields brothers they became very alarmed and made preparations to defend themselves against an attack, gathering their unsaddled horses around them on the top of a rise. Lewis sized up the situation. If he ran, the Indians would pursue, and Drewyer, alone in the valley, would be doomed. Putting on a bold front, Lewis advanced toward the Indians as one of them galloped full speed toward him. Lewis dismounted to show his lack of aggressive intent and waited for the Indian, who came close, took a look, and then returned to his friends. Soon a group of eight Indians approached. Lewis told the Fields brothers that these were Minnetares. In fact, the Indians were Piegan Blackfeet, the very tribe they did not want to encounter.

Lewis told his men they could expect to be robbed. If that happened he was prepared to defend himself to the death rather than have all his records and instruments stolen and destroyed. The Indians approached to within 100 yards, stopped, and one advanced to meet Lewis. Lewis told the Fields brothers to stand fast as he went to meet the solitary Indian. They shook hands. The ice had been broken, and the Indians invited Lewis to smoke with them. But he said that the man in the valley, Drewyer, had his pipe. The Indians, probably secretly convinced that they could over-power this small group whenever they wanted to, were agreeable that Drewyer should join the group.

When the party was reunited they went down into the valley to make a camp. The Indians set up a shelter, which they invited Lewis and his men to share with them. During the evening, and with Drewyer's help as interpreter, Lewis had a long conversation with the Indians. They were part of a large band camped some distance away, and there was a white man with them, presumably a British trader. The tribe was in the habit of traveling east to trade with the British, from whom they obtained rifles, ammunition, and whiskey in return for wolf and beaver skins.

Lewis turned on his charm. He told them where he had come from and that he had been to the ocean where the sun sets. He said that he had succeeded in restoring peace among the Indian tribes they had passed through, and that the Americans were going to set up trading posts that would supply the tribes with weapons and all the goods they desired. He wanted to give an impression of peace-ful strength. What he did not realize was that the Indians inter-preted his remarks in a different way. Here was a man who prided himself on uniting and arming the enemies of the Blackfeet. He was not a friend; he was a menace. The least they could do would be to steal his weapons.

Lewis and his men went to sleep, with Lewis taking the first watch. Early in the morning Joseph Fields was on guard and stupidly—or accidentally—laid down his weapon. One of the Indians crept up behind him and quietly pulled it away. Suddenly Joseph realized what was happening and all hell broke loose. The other Indians grabbed the guns beside Drewyer and Lewis and ran away. Reubin Fields quickly saw what was happening and, pulling his broad knife out of its scabbard, chased the man who had taken his gun. As he grappled with the thief, Fields plunged the knife into his chest. The man gasped once and died as Fields grabbed his rifle.

At this point Lewis woke from a deep sleep, found his rifle gone, and pulled out his pistol. Drewyer woke to find an Indian stealing his rifle. He wrestled with the man and pulled the rifle out of his hands. Two rifles stolen, two rifles quickly retrieved. Brandishing his pistol, Lewis chased and overtook the Indian who had stolen his rifle. The Fields brothers wanted to shoot the Indian, but Lewis ordered them not to. The Indian laid the rifle on the ground and walked away. Now it was three rifles stolen, three rifles retrieved.

At this point the Indians, having lost the weapons, decided they would steal the horses. Lewis and his men could not afford to have their horses stolen and chased the potential thieves. Lewis pursued two of the Indians and, when they had almost outrun him, ordered the Indian to release the horses. The Indian, hiding behind a rock, shouted at his friend who was nearby. Lewis, certain that the second man would attack him, fired and shot him through the gut, a fatal wound. The dying man turned, pointed his weapon at Lewis, and fired. The ball whistled over Lewis' head, the wind of the passing ball ruffling his hair.

Within seconds the tide of battle had turned. Lewis and his men had both their weapons and their horses. They had even more. They had all the Indians' horses, and their enemies were fleeing, leaving one dead and one fatally wounded behind them. Lewis threw the Indian shields and weapons on the fire and hung a medal around the neck of the dead man to tell the survivors who had done the deed.

As quickly as they could, Lewis and the men gathered the strongest horses, saddled and packed them, and galloped off. The ride of Paul Revere has rightly gone down in history, but compared with the next few hours, his ride was a short race. Within the next twenty-four hours Lewis and his men, mounted on good horses they had taken from the Indians, rode 120 miles, only resting themselves and the horses for a few hours in the early hours of the morning. As they approached the Missouri, Lewis was still not sure that all would be well and, again, said to his men that if they were attacked, they would sell their lives at the highest price. They did not have to pay the ultimate price because, as they got near the river, they heard the sound of shots fired by their own men coming down the river. "We quickly repaired to the joyfull sound . . . and had the unspeakable satisfaction to see our canoes coming down." Lady Luck was working overtime again.

Lewis opened the cache they had buried many months before and quickly retrieved what was salvageable. After they had been joined by Sergeant Gass and Willard, who had ridden down from the Great Falls, they canoed about 15 miles down the river and set up camp on the southern shore, putting the river between them and any followers. They dined sumptuously on bighorn sheep.

Lewis expressed no concerns in his journal about the fight with the Blackfeet that he had survived by the skin of his teeth. Before the voyage, people had expressed concern about Lewis' sometimes precipitate judgment. This incident was a prime example. Having decided to split the group at Traveler's Rest, he then divided it again into even weaker groups in order to penetrate the heart of Blackfeet territory. He was asking for trouble and found it.

Heavy rain fell for several days, and the group was lucky to find some old Indian houses in which to shelter. They made good time down the river. The water was thick with mud from the runoff and unpleasant to drink. A large bear came within 50 yards of the camp, stood on its hind legs to get a better sense of the visitors, and was immediately shot. "We fleeced it and extracted several gallons of oil." Later that day they killed an elk and four deer, calling into doubt Lewis' earlier statement that they only killed what they needed for food. In the previous few days they had killed nine bighorn sheep one day, seven more a day later, an elk, two beaver, and two bears. On August 3, the Fields brothers killed twenty-five deer. Lewis remarked that, "Deer are very abundant in the timbered bottoms of the river and are very gentle." Some of the animals killed were kept as specimens, although none were new species. Surrounded as they were by countless numbers of animals, there was no compunction to conserve. Even Lewis admitted that their attitude had changed. "In short, game is so abundant and gentle that we kill it when we please." They no longer thought of killing only what they needed.

The Missouri River was as treacherous as ever. Rounding a bend, one of the canoes went under an overhanging sweeper, and Willard was thrown overboard. Ordway, still aboard the canoe, drifted downstream for half a mile before he could land on the bank and go back to see what had happened to Willard, who was still clinging to the tree. Luckily, he was one of the stronger swimmers and was able to find two large branches to support him while he drifted downstream for a mile to a place where he could be rescued.

Men in ones and twos were constantly going off to hunt on their own. Colter and Collins went hunting on August 3 and did not return on time. Whenever men did not return as expected there was concern about their fate. Bands of Indians, some unfriendly, were never far away. By August 9, Colter and Collins still had not returned. "I fear some misfortune has happened them for their previous fidelity and orderly deportment induces me to believe that they would not thus intentionally delay." Lewis called a halt for two days to dress skins and make new clothes, to repair the pirogue that was leaking, and to wait for the hunters. Colter and Collins rejoined the others, none the worse, after an absence of nine days. The weather was terrible: rain, winds, lightning. The men were always wet and there was little protection for their things in the canoes. They were, however, making rapid progress. On August 7, Lewis hoped to cover 83 miles to reach the mouth of the Yellowstone and meet up with Clark. They achieved their aim, and at 4:00 P.M. went ashore at the mouth of the Yellowstone to find a note from Clark saying that he had already passed several days before. A few miles farther down were the remains of a recently vacated camp, with a fire still blazing and part of a hat that was recognized as belonging to Gibson. Clark and his party could not be far away.

On August 11, Lewis stopped to take some observations of the sun's meridian. While trying to do this he saw a herd of elk and went after it, taking Cruzatte with him. They killed one elk and wounded another, and both men went into the willows after the wounded animal. Lewis was about to fire when he was suddenly struck on the left thigh and both buttocks by a shot that penetrated his soft tissues but did not hit any bone or vital artery. He immediately thought, correctly, that Cruzatte—who was blind in one eye and had poor sight in the other—had shot him. Both of them were dressed in brown elk-skin clothes. They were an accident waiting to happen.

"Damn you, you've shot me," cried Lewis. There was no reply from Cruzatte, so Lewis thought that an Indian had shot him. He ran back to the pirogue, shouting to Cruzatte to watch out for the Indians and calling the others to arms. "I have been shot by an Indian, but I think I will live. Follow me. We've got to rescue Cruzatte." And they plunged back into the willows. After 100 yards Lewis' wounds hurt so badly he had to stop, and he ordered the men to keep going but to retreat under fire if they thought they were being overpowered.

Memories of the Marias and the Blackfeet must have been flashing through Lewis' mind. Good God! Have we come this far to be slaughtered just as success is around the corner? Twenty minutes later all worries were laid to rest. There were no Indians, and a crestfallen Cruzatte had been found. He claimed to have shot an elk after they had separated and had never heard Lewis shouting to him. Lewis, perhaps displaying some paranoia, concluded that Cruzatte had not shot him intentionally. Lewis took off his clothes and dressed the wounds himself, putting "tents" (drains) of lint into the entrance and exit wounds. He had bled considerably, but no vital structure had been damaged. He found the bullet in his breeches. When he had finished dressing his wounds he ordered the men to go and bring in the meat of the two elk that had been shot.

Lewis was made as comfortable as possible in the pirogue and tried to rest there all night, although in great pain and with a fever. They continued down the river the next morning and met two white trappers, Joseph Dickson and Forrest Hancock, the first white men they had seen since leaving Fort Mandan. They were headed up the Missouri, hunting unsuccessfully for beaver, and had met Clark the previous day.

On August 12, the Corps of Discovery was reunited. "At 1 P.M. I overtook Capt. Clark and party and had the pleasure of finding them all well." A quiet statement to record what must have been a moment of great relief and happiness, an exchange of stories, loud greetings, backslapping, and merriment.

Lewis, still in considerable pain, wrote in his journal that he would write no more until he recovered, and would leave to Clark the duty of keeping the record of the journey. He had done this several times before without such good reason, but this day was the last entry by Lewis. A botanist to the finish, he ended two years of writing with a description of the pin cherry. Clark examined and dressed Lewis' wounds and took over their care during the next days and weeks. The wounds healed before they reached St. Louis, and Lewis was not left with any residual disability. If the outcome had not been so happy, and Lewis had died at once from the wound or a subsequent infection, his legacy would have remained unchanged. His place in history was already assured.

Lewis and Clark had separated at Traveler's Rest on July 3, and reunited on August 12. During those weeks Clark rode to the Three Forks of the Missouri and then, across what is now Bozeman Pass, to the Yellowstone River. His group had an easier time than did Lewis and his men. He had no deadly encounters with Indians, although his party almost had all their horses stolen. He explored the Yellowstone River and a new route through the mountains. In his quiet way he had accomplished more than Lewis, for the Yellowstone would later become one of the major routes into the Rockies.

Clark's route lay through beautiful country with plenty of game for food and grazing for the horses. The first day out Potts fell ill "owing to riding a hard trotting horse." The cure was a pill of opium. Perhaps the problem was a painful rear end, rubbed sore from the trotting of the horse.

They made good progress, covering 30 miles on the second day. Signs of Indian scouts were everywhere. Within a few days the Indians made their presence known by stealing nine of the expedition's best horses. Not only were the Indians silent thieves, but they took the best horses. Clark ordered extra precautions. The horses would be hobbled and a sentry must inspect them after moonrise.

Clark wanted to follow a route described by the Shoshones, which was easier than the one they had taken the previous year. Sacagawea knew where they were and was able to point out the correct path. (This was one of the few occasions on which Sacagawea truly acted as a guide.) "The Indian woman," Clark wrote, "who has been of great service to me as a pilot through this country recommends a gap in the mountains more South which I will cross. . . ." His trust in Sacagawea was not misplaced, for this turned out to be an easy, direct, two-day route to the Yellowstone.

Most of the men were confirmed tobacco users, and one of the objectives they looked forward to was opening the cache that contained it. When the cache was reached the men could not wait. Some barely took time to take the saddles off their horses before reaching for the chewing tobacco that had been buried for months.

Although the month was July, the weather was cold and there was frost on the grass in the mornings. One night Clark laid out a basin of water, and, in the morning, it was covered with three-quarters of an inch of ice.

One morning Charbonneau went chasing buffalo on horseback and, when his horse stepped in a badger hole, was thrown, badly bruising his hip and shoulder. A day later Gibson was mounting his horse when he fell on a sharp snag that penetrated his thigh. He slept very little that night because of the pain and swelling extending from his hip to his knee. The wound became so painful that he could not ride longer than an hour and a half at a time. Clark ordered him to rest with Sergeant Pryor and follow later to the camp. A day later he was much better and the wound had obviously not become infected.

On July 24, 1806, the group separated again. Pryor and his men left to ride across the plains, while Clark loaded the canoes and set off down the Yellowstone River. Sergeant Pryor was given fourteen horses to travel overland to the Mandan village, where he would meet with Mr. Heney, an agent of the North West Company. As Pryor rode across the plains he passed herds of buffalo. Some of the horses with him were loose and carrying packs. When the loose horses saw the buffalo their Indian training came to the surface, and they immediately galloped off around the herd like equine herding dogs rounding up a flock of sheep. Pryor's solution was to have someone ride ahead and scare the buffalo away before the horses could see them.

For Clark's party, the current was rapid and they covered 70 miles the first day. One evening, off to the south, Clark saw a rocky prominence 200 feet high, which he climbed, and from which he got a fine view. He named the rock Pompey's Tower. Pompey was the nickname Clark had given Baptiste for whom he had developed a great fondness. Before Clark went back to camp he scratched his name and date on the rock. The tower is still a prominent monument and is the site of the only direct relic of the expedition; and Clark's signature can still be seen scratched into the rock. The trip down the Yellowstone was a wonderful experience. Game was plentiful. The scenery was interesting, and the river navigable without difficulty. There were few hazards, although Clark was nearly bitten by a rattlesnake. Most of the entries in the journal were descriptions of the land and its geology. Gibson still had some problems with his leg, but he was eventually able to walk normally.

The buffalo were breeding, and the males were making so much noise at night that they had to be chased away so the group could get some sleep. Bears sometimes came closer than was safe, partly because they could smell the meat that the men always carried on the canoes. The same rainstorms that made life miserable for Lewis after he regained the Missouri also soaked Clark and his party, causing him to complain that his situation was "a very disagreeable one. In an open canoe wet and without a possibility of keeping myself dry."

On August 8, to Clark's surprise, Sergeant Pryor and his party reappeared, without their horses, sailing down the river in buffalo-hide canoes. Two nights after leaving Clark, Pryor's group camped where there was good grass. The following morning, all the horses had been stolen. The tracks of the thieves came to within 100 yards of the camp, and the men followed them for 5 miles before realizing that the horses were gone for good. Being ingenious, reliant men, they made two small, round boats out of willow wands and buffalo hides. Also, being foresighted, they made two coracles in case one sank and they lost all their guns and ammunition.

The night after the horses were stolen Sergeant Pryor was bitten on the hand by a wolf while he was asleep. The wolf also attacked Richard Windsor and was shot by Shannon. This was a strange attack, because wolf attacks against humans have been extremely rare in North America. The wolf may have been rabid, but neither Pryor nor Windsor developed rabies. Perhaps it was sniffing around the sleeping men on the ground when Pryor moved his hand and the wolf responded by grabbing it. The smell of the men must have intrigued the wolf, and if Pryor had cleaned a deer that evening, there might still have been blood on his hand, attracting the wolf to investigate. Pryor's hand was not seriously harmed, suggesting that the wolf was inquisitive rather than aggressive. If the wolf had been aggressive, there would not have been much left of Pryor's hand.

When Clark's party reached the junction of the Yellowstone and the Missouri the mosquitoes were so bad that the men could not camp there. So, after leaving a message for Lewis, they continued on down the Missouri. A day later they reunited with Lewis and found their Captain languishing in his pirogue with gunshot wounds.

There were many miles to go, but the men were headed downstream, and the speed of the current swept them along at a brisk rate. Lewis' wound was the main source of worry. Infection was a serious risk, and Clark looked at the wound anxiously every day when he dressed it. Although healing was slow, no serious complications arose. By the time the journey came to an end Lewis had recovered entirely.

After leaving the Yellowstone, there were visits to make at the villages of the Mandans and the Minnetares. The Mandan Chief was delighted to see them again but complained that he did not have enough corn and that the Teton Sioux had been very troublesome. He was afraid to accompany the party back to Washington because he would have to pass the Sioux along the way. Clark tried to persuade some of the Indians to go with them to Washington to "see their Great Father and hear his good words and receive his bountiful gifts." There were no takers except one young man whom they knew to be a troublemaker and who had already stolen a knife belonging to one of Clark's party. It was grudgingly returned, but the man was not taken down the river.

The end of the expedition was in sight. Colter had no desire to return to civilization. He wanted to go back to the mountains and hunt for beaver with some other trappers who had made him a good offer. The big city held no attraction for him. He was given his release, provided no other military personnel asked for the same privilege. All agreed to stay to the end. The agreement did not extend to Charbonneau and his family. Charbonneau did not think he could make a living as an interpreter lower down the river and elected to stay in the Mandan village. Clark offered to take Baptiste, "a butifull promising child," but both Charbonneau and Sacagawea were unwilling to let him go until he had been weaned. He was nineteen months old. In a year he would be old enough to leave his mother, and they would be happy to bring him then if Clark was willing to raise him. Clark agreed.

Although, overall, little was mentioned of them in the journals, Clark wrote more about Sacagawea and Baptiste than did Lewis. Some imaginative authors have suggested there was romance between Clark and Sacagawea, but there is not the slightest evidence for this. Clark liked the little boy and, in subsequent years supported him well.

On the way north in the first year of the voyage the Teton Sioux had tried their best to cause trouble. Lewis and Clark had no desire to get into an argument with them again. When they once more passed through their territory they were constantly on guard and made sure that their weapons were in working order.

The Corps met the Teton Sioux on August 30. Ninety men appeared on the bank of the river armed with bows and guns. They fired some guns as a salute, but when Clark sent someone to inquire who they were and found that they were the Sioux, he did not want to deal with them. He told them that they were bad people and no white traders would come to them again because they had treated others so badly. They were warned not go to war with the Mandans, who had been well armed with weapons from the expedition. Lewis and Clark had given the Mandans the old blunderbuss, and perhaps this knowledge would deter the Sioux from attacking them. The confrontation ended with the Sioux shouting abuse and making rude gestures from the bank as the canoes slipped down the stream. The expedition was glad to get by without violence.

The last three weeks of the voyage went by without trouble. At one place there was shooting near the river, and Lewis hobbled up on the bank to find out what was happening. It turned out that the firing came from some Indians who were shooting at an old keg. Young men shooting at beer cans is an age-old sport.

Lewis' gunshot wound improved steadily. On September 4, Lewis, Clark, and some of the men climbed the bluff overlooking the river where Sergeant Floyd had been buried. The grave had been partially opened by the Indians, so the men filled it in again. Later stories suggested that a Chief had wanted his son to be buried with Floyd and acquire some of his power. When the grave was moved, years later, no evidence of two sets of bones could be found. The entry in Clark's journal was brief and to the fact, but as the men stood there they must have blessed their good fortune in not losing any more men. There was not much sickness in the last part of the journey. Clark became ill and directed that a pint of chocolate be made, which he drank with great relief for whatever symptoms he had. Many of the men suffered again from eyes irritated by dust and sun. Travelers going up the river generously gave them whiskey and pork, which they had not tasted in many months. The effect of the whiskey and the thoughts of soon arriving home raised morale. "Our party received a dram and sung songs untill 11o'clock at night in the greatest harmony."

A few days before reaching their final destination Captain Robert McClellan, formerly of the Artillery, who was embarking on a speculative business endeavor, hoping to make his way overland to trade with the Spanish, met them on the river. He was astonished to see them, for most people, except for the optimistic President, thought the expedition had perished. McClellan also brought the men up-to-date on the political situation and gave them biscuits, chocolate, sugar, and more whiskey.

As they neared St. Louis, three men could not row because of the state of their eyes, so Clark consolidated the crews into fewer boats. Two days away from St. Louis, their spirits were raised by seeing cows. The people of St. Charles, dressed in their Sunday finery, who had waved good-bye to them so many months before, came pouring out to welcome them into their homes. The hospitality for men supposed to be long since dead knew no bounds.

At 12 noon on Thursday, September 23, 1806, the Corps of Discovery reached St. Louis. They fired off their guns in salute. The news of their approach had spread quickly through the village (St. Louis was hardly a town yet), and all the people ran down to the river to see the men who had traveled to the setting sun and returned. The transformation from frontier adventurers to officers of the town was rapid. "We payed a friendly visit to (Mes. Choteau and) Mr (Ogustus) August Choteau and some of our old friends this evening." The next morning Clark wrote that he had slept little the night before. Sleeping in a bed with sheets was a strange feeling, and he must have spent long hours staring at the ceiling, marveling at what they had seen and done. On September 25, the citizens of St. Louis gave them a dinner and ball at William Christy's Tavern. Eighteen toasts were drunk, the last to "Captains Lewis and Clark—Their perilous services endear them to every American heart."

NINE

Afterthoughts:
Doctors in Today's Wilderness

The cottonwoods were beginning to turn, splotches of gold against the green of a departing summer, when Lewis and the Corps of Discovery pulled into the shore at St. Louis at noon on September 23, 1806. A short distance upstream from the town they fired off their rifles and the jubilant townsfolk came running down to the river's edge to meet them. There was cheering and shouting, backslapping and handshaking. The canoes were pulled up on the shore and ready hands helped the Corps unload and carry their gear to William Christy's storeroom. Lewis and Clark were invited to stay with Peter Choteau, a local businessman. Water was heated for a bath and a shave and, somewhere, new clothes were found and, perhaps, the travel-worn elk-skin pants with a bullet hole in the seat were shown to their host, amidst laughter, before being thrown out the back door. In the afternoon, after a hurried note had been dispatched to John Hay, the post-master at Cahokia, asking him to delay the post, Lewis sat down and wrote to the President.

The letter to the President was not tinged with doubt. It was a simple, straightforward account of what had been accomplished. Lewis concentrated on the commercial implications of what they had seen and done. He confirmed what Jefferson wanted to hear, that the fur trade would be easier along the new route and would give quick access to the rich trade of China. As a postscript to the letter, Lewis added, perhaps belatedly, "N.B. The whole of the party who accompanied me from the Mandans have returned in good health, which is not, I assure you, to me one of the least pleasing considerations of the voyage."

Lewis could not know that history would show that he had failed to find the best route to the West. All he knew was that he had followed his President's orders and had returned, successful. It does not matter that the route he followed did not become the major road to the West Coast, or that years had to pass before the Oregon Trail was opened in 1842 and thousands of settlers made their way to the Promised Land. Lewis was assured of his achievement, and his accomplishments stand alone today.

Organizing an expedition, like the Lewis and Clark journey to the Pacific, in modern times would be a huge undertaking and a much more complicated task than it was in 1803. First, it would be hard to find an area of the world in which an expedition could travel for two years through a land without cities—with only a scattered, primitive population. A route might be found in some parts of Australia, the North Pole, northern Russia, Antarctica, or in outer space; but the exact conditions of travel could not be duplicated. Clothes, weapons, food, transportation, camping equipment, medicines, and surgical supplies would be radically different from the elk-skin clothes, the buffalo meat, the canoes carved from cottonwood trees, and the leaking tents endured by the Corps of Discovery.

It is interesting to wonder what Meriwether Lewis would buy if he was resurrected and had to go shopping for a modern expedition. Certainly clothing made of high-tech materials; but what would happen to them after they wore out in a year and there was no one to repair them or make clothes from animal skins? The weapons would of course be more accurate and more powerful. But would there be a gunsmith who could fire up the furnace and make spare parts in camp from scrap metal found on the trail? Nowhere in the world would it be possible, or allowable, to shoot enough animals to provide meat for more than thirty men for two years. Taking enough food for the group would be a major problem. Not many people would like to be asked to select food for two years for thirty men with different appetites and tastes. Expeditions to Mount Everest spend a lot of money and time choosing food (as did Lewis and Clark) that will be tasty and nutritious, but even now, occasional mistakes are made, such as the time only pumpernickel bread was brought for an international expedition. In days when soldiers did not eat Meals Ready to Eat but had to accept salt meat and stale vegetables, the pounds of buffalo, elk, and deer the men of the Corps often ate were better than most camp food.

The modern boats chosen for a river expedition would most likely be rubber rafts with outboard motors: convenient, powerful, with a shallow draft, but very heavy to portage. They could be rowed and dragged upstream and would be lighter than a keelboat, but it would be impossible to carry enough fuel for the length of the trip. Prearranged caches or airlifts would be essential.

Visas for all the countries to be visited, as well as climbing permits, commercial endorsements, and funds would have to be obtained. Finally, everything would have to be collected in one place, at the right time, and shipped to the starting point—a doable task. Companies now organize outdoor expeditions and coordinate gear and permits for large groups. Numerous alliances, businesses, and governments continue to sponsor large exploratory expeditions. But almost nothing rivals the magnitude and duration of the Lewis and Clark expedition.

Furthermore, the medical aspects of exploration have matured greatly since 1804 and especially in the past thirty years. Charles Houston is an octogenarian who belies his age by two decades. He has been a doctor, world-class mountaineer, pioneer in altitude medicine, Peace Corps leader, and an occasional burr under the saddle of those who could not keep up with his imagination and drive. In 1975, he organized the first of several medical conferences on Mountain Medicine. Doctors, nurses, scientists, paramedics, and climbers gathered beneath the cliffs of the Yosemite valley to hear experts talk on heat and cold, first aid, trauma, search-and-rescue, and altitude sickness, emphasizing the management of injuries in distant places, and in areas where help is far away.

There had been other, smaller gatherings that discussed mountain medicine, and a book, *Medicine for Mountaineers*, was published in 1967. But the Yosemite meeting acted as a catalyst that started people thinking about mountain medicine as a unique body of knowledge. Soon, a new term was coined from the flood of emerging ideas, "Wilderness Medicine."

Wilderness Medicine has become a collecting house for knowledge about illnesses and accidents that affect the wilderness traveler: everything from heat exhaustion to heart attacks, bee stings to snakebites, lightning strikes to drowning. There are now professional societies devoted to the discipline that regularly hold educational conferences around the world. This compendium of knowledge has spawned textbooks and medical journals. What occurred on the Lewis and Clark expedition was the epitome of wilderness medicine: the provision of care in a remote place, with no hospital, no laboratory, no X-ray, CAT scan, or MRI. Just diagnoses made using only the natural senses, and care coming out of a backpack.

Nowadays, the doctors, paramedics, medical supplies, and equipment that accompany major expeditions are, of course, vastly different from those of 1804. Big expeditions take a doctor experienced in the problems of the environment the explorers will encounter: an expert in tropical medicine for a jungle journey, someone knowledgeable in high altitude for Everest, a specialist in baro-medicine for an ocean-diving expedition.

Planning the medical care for a large expedition is complicated and expensive. The members of the expedition have to be recruited and vetted medically. Their past medical histories have to be known and files kept on illnesses or accidents they have had in the past. Fear of having an attack of appendicitis while high on a mountain has persuaded occasional explorers to have their appendix removed voluntarily to prevent that possibility. Pre-expedition immunizations, dental exams and treatment, blood group identification, and knowledge of the health requirements and amenities of countries to be visited take time and effort. For instance, some countries demand specific inoculations for all entrants. No expedition wants to lose a member at the border because of lack of an immunization or other oversights.

The medical kit also requires careful planning. What will be the environment of the expedition? What are the likely medical emergencies? It is impossible to prepare for every problem and the doctor must be ready to improvise. Will there be a base camp and satellite camps? Will each camp require a separate medical kit? If so, how elaborate? Should every member carry their own medical kit, and what should it contain, apart from personal needs? How should the medical kit be packed? What is the medical expertise of other members of the expedition apart from the doctor, and how can it be used?

Lewis and Clark, with the aid of Benjamin Rush, prepared a medical kit that covered most of the problems they could foresee or reasonably deal with. There were almost no supplies for treating gunshot or arrow wounds that penetrated the body cavities because they knew they could not deal with them. The equipment now taken for massive trauma may only be sufficient to support the victims for a few hours until a helicopter whisks them away to a hospital. Operations are sometimes done under primitive circumstances when there is no alternative. Peter Steele, an English surgeon and climber, traveling by himself in a remote part of Nepal, once successfully operated on a local shepherd with a strangulated hernia, using morphine and liquor for anesthesia, and the needles and thread from his sewing kit. If he had walked away from the challenge the young man would have died.

The modern expedition doctor may have to prepare himself with skills he does not always use. Most expedition doctors, although skilled physicians, have no training in dental care before going on the expedition and would only extract a painful tooth under the most pressing circumstances. A few instructional sessions in a dentist's office may pay off handsomely months later. Also, not many doctors in the United States have ever seen a case of malaria, yet the expedition may have to go through an area in which malaria is endemic and virulent. Expedition doctors train to recognize and treat diseases and injuries with which they are not familiar but may encounter. Treating hypothermia, frostbite, snakebites, scorpion stings, and poisonous fish and jellyfish stings are not daily procedures for the average doctor, yet knowing how to deal with them might become a lifesaving necessity.

The medical kit that Lewis and Clark took contained thirty-two medications, many of them useless by modern standards. A modern expedition medical kit contains, at least, the following basic medications: antibiotics; pain killers from morphine to aspirin; drugs to deal with asthma and respiratory complications; cures for a serious nosebleed; eye medications for infections, snow blindness, and foreign bodies; sedatives and sleeping pills; medications for gastroenteritis and hemorrhoids; pills for altitude sickness (if going high); drugs and equipment for cardiac resuscitation; ointments for everything from insect bites to severe allergic reactions; supplies and instruments for dealing with lacerations, blisters, burns, and impaled foreign bodies; and supplies of intravenous fluids. An extreme high-altitude expedition should have a Gamow bag for rapid compression of someone with cerebral edema. The cost of modern kits runs into the thousands of dollars, but is frequently reduced by donations from drug and equipment suppliers. Bright yellow tents or windproof jackets with the name of the supplier on the side are great advertisements.

Not only are the supplies available now totally different—and more effective—than those that Lewis took, but the management and variety of the problems are different. Antibiotics could have shortened many of the infections that troubled the men on the river. Snakebite antivenin is available, but it would not have been used for the bites that Joseph Fields and others sustained—the bites were not severe enough. The most commonly available antivenin for North American snakes is derived from horse serum and causes many allergic reactions in the recipients. As a result, it is not used unless the bite is likely to produce serious damage or death.

Many of the eye problems that plagued the men of the Corps would have been prevented and treated better by modern methods.

Goggles protect eyes from flying dust, and sunglasses stop ultra-violet rays reflected off snow and river water. Most of the Indians' eye problems could now be treated easily. If Clark had been able to anticipate the number of natives with diseases of the eye, and the benefit the expedition would have received from treating them, he would probably have taken a larger supply of the ingredients for "eye water."

The journals of Lewis and Clark mention virtually nothing about camp sanitation, but plenty about diarrhea. Although they must have known that there was a connection between the two, diarrhea was not a subject worthy of discussion. Perhaps Lewis thought it an inappropriate subject for a document that would be given to the President. A modern expedition would be well sup-plied with large-capacity water filters and tablets for water purifi-cation. The frequent attacks of diarrhea that plagued the Lewis and Clark expedition could have been almost eliminated with better preventive precautions, but again, understanding of health in the nineteenth century did not allow for such conclusions. Treatment with antibiotics might have been only sometimes necessary, but the cure would have been effective and quick, and the lives of the men would have been more comfortable.

Considering the lack of care given to minor wounds and lacera-tions, the imbedded cactus spines, the abrasions and blisters that were a constant source of irritation, there were, surprisingly, few serious infections. Clark had to hobble around for a few days with a painful infection on his ankle, but Lewis and Gibson both escaped infectious complications of potentially serious penetrating wounds. When Lewis was shot he was fortunate that both the entrance and exit wounds were obvious and that the bullet ended up in his leather pants rather than in his buttock. If there had not been an exit wound, Clark might have felt compelled to try to extract the ball from the wound. Removal of the bullet was the standard practice of the day. An operation with unsterile instru-ments, probing deep into the soft tissues, would almost certainly have resulted in a serious infection. When Gibson fell off his horse on to a stick that penetrated his thigh, he was lucky that the wound did not become infected, because the only way to treat the infection, in the absence of antibiotics, would have been to open and drain it—a skill that Clark did not have.

The lack of serious complications of the wounds and illnesses that occurred is a tribute to the recuperative powers of the human body, healing powers that are sometimes ignored or forgotten nowadays. Many of the wounds would certainly now be treated with antibiotics, but the results with the men of the Corps showed that it was possible to get better without treatment, perhaps slower and with more discomfort, but the results were the same.

When Lewis was planning the expedition he did not anticipate having a young woman and a child as members of the Corps. Imagine a modern polar or Everest expedition with a young girl carrying an infant strapped to her back. But Lewis was not the only explorer in history to deal with this dilemma. Samuel Hearne, venturing up the Coppermine River in northern Canada in 1767, faced the same situation. An Indian woman with his group delivered a child after "having suffered the birth pangs for fifty-two hours." As soon as she was delivered "the poor creature then took her infant on her back and set out with the rest of our company."

Although Lewis says nothing about it in his journal, he presumably assumed that Sacagawea and her husband would take care of any problems that might arise with the baby. There was no alternative source of food for the infant other than breast milk, and it would have been several months before Baptiste could possibly have taken any solid food. This worry does not seem to have crossed Lewis' mind. He had sympathy for Sacagawea when she became sick, but he seemed to have almost as much concern for losing her as an interpreter as for losing her as a person.

Lewis' concern over Clark being seen as a doctor obviously reflects his innate honesty. He had tried hard to be honest in his other relations with the Indians and had been telling them in his speeches that white people could be trusted. The deception of suggesting that Clark was a doctor obviously worried him. The modern doctor, traveling as an expedition medical officer or as an individual, faces similar problems of conscience. The doctor will always be called on to help the local people, whether they are the sick villagers, or local porters and workers employed by the expedition. In his account of climbing Annapurna in 1951, Maurice Herzog wrote about the relation between the expedition doctor, Jacques Oudot, and the Nepalese villagers: "Oudot had tremendous prestige. People came long distances to see him, for he had become a sort of god. We admired the touching simplicity of these creatures who put their health and sometimes their lives in the hands of a complete stranger."

Most countries now have a health-care system of some sort, even if it is scattered and not very efficient. Providing care that the local system cannot may be beneficial to individuals but can undermine their confidence in the established clinics. Lewis and Clark were lucky, the local medicine men were the only rival system, and they did not object to the ministrations of Clark. If the medicine men were upstaged and annoyed, their reactions did not get into the journals. Mostly the local Chiefs welcomed, and used, the services Clark provided. Clark was fortunate that none of the Indians he treated died. "Do no harm" is an overriding principle, and sometimes, even today, the best way to follow this is to do nothing.

Wilderness medicine has certainly changed over time, especially with advanced methods of communication and transportation. Detailed plans are now made for the evacuation of seriously ill or injured expedition members. Lewis and Clark's only contingency plan was to appoint the next in command. Evacuation procedures were never a realistic possibility for the Corps. Today, however, the availability of care combined with the use of sophisticated communication systems and aircraft make evacuation feasible and efficacious, especially from remote areas. Unfortunately, these services are often only available to members of the expedition and not to the native population. For Lewis and Clark, evacuation was possible but only by the long and hazardous return route down the river. When Sacagawea was very sick at the Great Falls

Charbonneau wanted to return to the Mandan village. This was not a ridiculous request. Lewis had even considered sending back a party with news and specimens after they had reached the Great Falls. But, wisely, he did not want to divide the group, because there were not enough men in the party for safety. Charbonneau's request was refused.

No expedition in North America has received closer scrutiny and brought greater rewards than that of Lewis and Clark. They catalogued the American West—its landscapes, flora and fauna, and peoples. Their efforts still carry an aura of valiant achievement, and thousands of supporters keep the memories bright and the hero worship alive through historical organizations, preservation of the expedition's trail, countless books, conventions, and promotions. The Lewis and Clark expedition continues to be a testament for exploration.

It was an enormous achievement to take a group of more than thirty men, plus a woman and an infant, across an uncharted continent, let alone to return with only one death. This could only be achieved with great leadership, wonderful organization, or unending luck. Lewis and Clark were admired, perhaps even loved, by their men, who regarded the Captains as tough but compassionate leaders. Lewis was an active leader, who maintained his authority and yet also took time and effort to work alongside his men. Many other exploratory expeditions without such leadership have fallen apart.

Planning, leadership, and selection of skilled and able men, combined with discipline, loyalty, and luck—lots of luck—held the Corps of Discovery together. Many expeditions have overcome greater hazards, survived worse weather, and endured prolonged starvation but achieved far less. The measure of the Corps' success owes itself in part to the lack of disasters. Mountains were climbed, plains were crossed, rivers and rapids were run. The men came through the challenges unscathed. The men of the Corps certainly sensed that they were doing something special, but they had no vision of how their success would open a continent and build a nation. They regarded themselves as ordinary men doing what they had volunteered to do. When all was finished they dispersed and most were never heard from again. There were no reunions, no annual dinners, and newsletters. They simply took their pay and their land grants. Some of them married, some turned around and went back up the river, some fought in wars, some went home to jobs and farms. Some died fighting, some died in their beds, some died unknown. Within days of reaching St. Louis, they took a last drink together, bid farewell, and returned to their lives.

When Lewis sat down to write to the President on that September afternoon in St. Louis, he may have paused, wondering how to begin. He dipped his quill pen in the ink and wrote,

> Sir, It is with pleasure that I announce to you the safe arrival of myself and party at 12 o'clock today at this place with our papers and baggage. In obedience to your orders we have penetrated the Continent of North America to the Pacific Ocean, and sufficiently explored the interior of the country to affirm with confidence that we have discovered the most practicable rout which dose exist across the continent by means of the navigable branches of the Missouri and Columbia Rivers.

Orders fulfilled. Mission accomplished.

Appendix A

Members of the Corps of Discovery

A. The following went from the Mandan village to the Pacific Ocean and back.

Capt. Meriwether Lewis
Capt. William Clark
York, Clark's servant
Sgt. Patrick Gass
Sgt. John Ordway
Sgt. Nathaniel Pryor
Pvt. William Bratton
Pvt. John Collins
Pvt. John Colter
Pvt. Peter Cruzatte
Pvt. Joseph Fields
Pvt. Reuben Fields
Pvt. Robert Frazier
Pvt. George Gibson
Pvt. Silas Goodrich
Pvt. Hugh Hall
Pvt. Thomas Proctor Howard
Pvt. Francois Labiche
Pvt. Jean Baptiste LePage

Pvt. Hugh McNeal
Pvt. John Potts
Pvt. George Shannon
Pvt. John Shields
Pvt. John B. Thompson
Pvt. Peter M. Weiser
Pvt. William Werner
Pvt. Joseph Whitehouse
Pvt. Alexander Hamilton Willard
Pvt. Richard Windsor
George Drouillard (Drewyer), interpreter and hunter
Toussaint Charbonneau, interpreter
Jean Baptiste Charbonneau, Sacagawea and Charbonneau's son
Sacagawea, Charbonneau's wife

B. The following joined at the Mandan village.

Jean Baptiste Charbonneau
Toussaint Charbonneau
Phillipe Degis
Pierre Dorion, Sr.

Joseph Gravelines
Pvt. Jean Baptiste Lepage
Sacagawea

C. The following served only from St. Louis to the Mandan village and returned after the winter of 1804–1805.

Sgt. Charles Floyd, died 8/20/04

Cpl. John Boley

Cpl. John Dame

Cpl. Jean Baptiste DeChamps

Cpl. John Newman
(court-martialed)

Cpl. John G. Robertson

Cpl. Ebenezer Tuttle

Cpl. Richard Warfington
(commander of return group)

Cpl. Isaac White

Pvt. Joseph Barter,
"La Liberté" (deserted)

Pvt. Moses B. Reed
(dishonorably discharged)

Engagés:

Alexander Carson

Charles Caugee

Joseph Collin

Pierre Roi

Charles Hebert

Jean Baptiste LaJeunnesse

Étienne Malboeuf

Peter Pinaut

Paul Primeau

Francois Rivet

Roky

Appendix B

What Happened Afterward?

CAPT. MERIWETHER LEWIS (1774–1809): Appointed Governor of the Louisiana Territory after the expedition. Died by his own hand in a small inn in Natchez, Tennessee, while on his way to Washington, D.C. He had experienced political and personal problems. Some people believe he was murdered, but there is no categorical evidence to support this opinion.

SECOND LT. (CAPT.) WILLIAM CLARK (1770–1838): Appointed Governor of the Missouri Territory and was responsible for relations with the Indians. He took Baptiste Charbonneau under his care and ensured that he was educated.

SGT. PATRICK GASS (1771–1804): Remained in the Army and fought in the War of 1812 and accidentally lost an eye. Retired to a small farm and married, at sixty, to a sixteen-year-old girl, Maria Hamilton. He was the longest living survivor of the Corps of Discovery.

SGT. JOHN ORDWAY (1775–1817?): Went to Washington with Lewis after the expedition to accompany an Indian chief. Settled in Missouri, married. Date of death is uncertain.

SGT. NATHANIEL HALE PRYOR (1772–1831): In 1807 was responsible for returning Sheheke to his home village, but had to turn back because of Arikara opposition. Rejoined the Army and rose to rank of Captain. Married an Osage woman. The town of Pryor, Montana, is named after him.

PVT. WILLIAM E. BRATTON (1778–1841): Lived in Kentucky and fought in the War of 1812. Married in 1819. Is buried in Waynetown, Indiana.

PVT. JOHN COLLINS (?–1823): Died while on a trapping expedition with William Ashley to the upper Missouri: killed by Arikara Indians.

PVT. JOHN COLTER (1775–1813): Left the expedition at the Mandan village and returned to the mountains. Became one of the most famous Mountain Men, and is well known for an adventurous escape from Blackfeet Indians. The first white man to see the geysers of Yellowstone.

PVT. PIERRE CRUZATTE (dates uncertain): May have gone on John McClellan's expedition to the Rockies in 1807. Cause of death unknown.

INTERPRETER GEORGE DROUILLARD (DREWYER) (?–1810): Returned to fur trading with Manuel Lisa and died in a battle with Blackfeet in 1810.

PVTS. JOSEPH (1772–1807) and REUBEN FIELDS (1771–1823): Joseph was killed a year after the expedition, perhaps while serving with John McClellan. Reuben married, settled in Kentucky, and died in 1823.

PVT. ROBERT FRAZIER (?–1837): Went with Lewis to Washington, returned to Missouri where he died.

PVT. GEORGE GIBSON (?–1809): Was perhaps with Pryor trying to return Sheheke to the Mandans. Died in St. Louis.

PVT. GEORGE SHANNON (1785–1836): Wounded in a battle with the Arikara while trying to return Sheheke to the Mandans; wounded and lost a leg; helped Nicholas Biddle edit the journals of the expedition; studied law; and served as a Senator from Missouri.

PVT. JOHN SHIELDS (1769–1809): expert gunsmith, became a trapper with Daniel Boone, a relative. Settled and died in Indiana.

BAPTISTE CHARBONNEAU (1804–1866): Was adopted by Clark, educated, became the ward of Prince Paul of Würtemberg, went to Europe for some years, and returned to the United States. He became a hunting guide, but eventually went to California where he died.

TOUSSAINT CHARBONNEAU (dates uncertain): After the expedition he lived with Indian tribes. The Mandans were decimated by smallpox in 1837. Charbonneau was known to be alive and in his eighties in 1839.

SACAGAWEA (dates uncertain): accompanied Baptiste to St. Louis while he was being educated. There are two stories about her death. The most likely is that she died of a "putrid fever" in 1812. The other story is that she lived to an old age and died on a reservation and is buried near Lander, Wyoming. There is a grave with her name on it, but there is some doubt about the origin of the person buried there. There are two markers beside her grave, one for Basil, another son, and one for Baptiste.

YORK (1770–?): Clark's slave. Received his freedom around 1811 and operated a freight business. The details of his death are uncertain. He may have died from cholera in 1832 or in the Rockies with the Crows.

Bibliography

Annotated references have not been included in the text because this book is intended for the general reader, rather than for the historian. All the quotations from the journals of Lewis, Clark, and others have been taken from volumes 2–11 of *The Journals of the Lewis and Clark Expedition*, edited by Gary Moulton and published by the University of Nebraska Press. The other books and scientific papers listed were all used in the preparation of the manuscript and are a mine of information, ready to be explored by any reader who wants to dig deeper into the wonderful story of Lewis and Clark.

BOOKS

Allen, John Logan. *Lewis and Clark and the Image of the American Northwest.* New York: Dover Publications, 1975.

Ambrose, Stephen E. *Undaunted Courage.* New York: Simon and Schuster, 1996.

———. *Comrades.* New York: Simon and Schuster, 1999.

Bakeless, John, ed. *The Journals of Lewis and Clark.* Mentor Books, 1964.

Barth, Gunther, ed. *The Lewis and Clark Expedition. Selections from the Journals Arranged by Topic.* Bedford, Mass.: St. Martin's, 1998.

Binger, Carl. *Revolutionary Doctor: Benjamin Rush 1746–1813.* New York: W. W. Norton, 1966.

Botkin, Daniel B. *Our Natural History: The Lessons of Lewis and Clark.* New York: Perigee Books, 1995.

———. *Passage of Discovery; The American Rivers Guide to the Missouri River of Lewis and Clark.* New York: Perigee Books, 1999.

Carpenter, Kenneth J. *The History of Scurvy & Vitamin C.* Cambridge, England: Cambridge University Press, 1986.

Chuinard, Eldon G., M.D. *Only One Man Died.* Fairfield, Wash.: Ye Galleon Press, 1999.

Clark, Ella E. and Margot Edmonds. *Sacagawea of the Lewis and Clark Expedition.* Berkeley: University of California Press, 1979.

Coues, Elliot, ed. *The History of the Lewis and Clark Expedition*, vols. 1–3. New York: Dover Publications. Reprint of 1893 volumes. 1999.

Cutright, Paul Russell. *Lewis and Clark: Pioneering Naturalists.* Lincoln: University of Nebraska Press, 1969.

Desowitz, Robert S., M.D. *The Malaria Capers. More Tales of Parasites, People, Research and Reality.* New York: W. W. Norton, 1991.

———. *Who Gave Pinta to the Santa Maria? Torrid Diseases in a Temperate World.* New York: W. W., 1997.

de Voto, Bernard, ed. *The Journals of Lewis and Clark.* Boston: Houghton Mifflin. Reprint. 1997.

de Voto, Bernard. *The Course of Empire.* Boston: Houghton Mifflin, 1998.

Dillon, Richard. *Meriwether Lewis.* Santa Cruz, Calif.: Western Tanager Press, 1988.

Duncan, Dayton. *Out West: American Journey along the Lewis and Clark Trail.* New York: Penguin Books, 1987.

Duncan, Dayton, and Ken Burns. *Lewis and Clark: The Journey of the Corps of Discovery.* New York: Alfred A. Knopf, 1997.

Friedman, Meyer, M.D., and Gerald Friedland. *Medicine's Ten Greatest Discoveries.* New Haven, Conn.: Yale University Press, 1998.

Furtwangler, Albert. *Acts of Discovery: Visions of America in the Lewis and Clark Journals.* Urbana: University of Illinois Press, 1999.

Goetzmann, William H., and Glyndwr Williams. *The Atlas of North American Exploration.* Norman: University of Oklahoma Press, 1992.

Gunther, Erna. *Ethnobotany of Western Washington.* Seattle: University of Washington Press, 1973.

Guthrie, Douglas. *A History of Medicine.* London: Thomas Nelson, & Son, 1945.

Harris, Burton. *John Colter: His Years in the Rockies.* Lincoln: University of Nebraska Press, 1993.

Jackson, Donald. *Letters of the Lewis and Clark Expedition*, with related documents. Urbana: University of Illinois Press, 1962.

———. *Thomas Jefferson and the Stony Mountains: Exploring the West from Monticello.* Urbana: University of Illinois Press, 1981.

Johnson, Paul. *A History of the American People.* New York: HarperCollins, 1997.

Jones, Landon Y. *The Essential Lewis and Clark.* New York: The Ecco Press, 2000

Jones, T. Wharton. *The Principles and Practice of Ophthalmic Medicine and Surgery*. Philadelphia: Lea and Blanchard, 1847.

Lamar, Howard R., ed. *The New Encyclopedia of the American West*. New Haven, Conn.: Yale University Press, 1998.

Leach, John. *Survival Psychology*. New York: New York University Press, 1994.

Macgregor, Carol Lynn, ed. *The Journals of Patrick Gass: Member of the Lewis and Clark Expedition*. Missoula, Montana: Mountain Press Publishing Company, 1997.

Mackenzie, Alexander. Walter Sheppe, ed.: *Journal of the Voyage to the Pacific*. New York: Dover Publications, 1995.

Montgomery, M. R. *Jefferson and the Gun-Men: How the West Was Almost Lost*. New York: Crown Publishers, 2000.

Moulton, Gary E., ed. *The Journals of the Lewis and Clark Expedition*, vols. 2–11. Lincoln: University of Nebraska 1997.

Norton, A. B., M.D. *Ophthalmic Disease and Therapeutics*, Philadelphia: Boericke and Tafel, 1892.

Onuf, Peter S. *Jefferson's Empire: The Language of American Nationhood*. Charlottesville: University Press of Virginia, 2000.

Porter, Roy, ed. *Cambridge Illustrated History of Medicine*. Cambridge, England: Cambridge University Press, 1996.

Ronda, James P. *Lewis and Clark among the Indians*. Lincoln: University of Nebraska Press, 1984.

Rubin, Rick. *Naked Against the Rain: The People of the Lower Columbia River*. Portland, Oreg.: Far Shore Press, 1999.

Schmidt, Thomas. *National Geographic Guide to the Lewis and Clark Trail*. Washington, D.C.: National Geographic Society, 1998.

Schneiders, Robert Kelley. *Unruly River: Two Centuries of Change along the Missouri*. Lawrence: University Press of Kansas, 1999.

Stevenson, Elizabeth. *Figures in a Western landscape*. Baltimore, Md.: Johns Hopkins University Press, 1994.

Strong, Emory and Ruth. *Seeking Western Waters*. Ed: Herbert K. Beals. Oregon Historical Society Press, 1995.

Townsend, John Kirk. *Narrative of a Journey: Across the Rocky Mountains to the Columbia River*. Introduction and Annotation by George A. Jobanek. Corvallis: Oregon State University Press, 1999.

Van der Linden, Frank. *The Turning Point: Jefferson's Battle for the Presidency*. Golden, Colo.: Fulcrum Publishing, 2000.

Vogel, Virgil J. *American Indian Medicine*. Norman: University of Oklahoma Press, 1970.

SCIENTIFIC PAPERS

Bates, D. G. Sydenham and the medical meaning of "method." *Bull. Hist. Med.* 51: 324–338. 1977.

Bowers J. Z. The odyssey of smallpox vaccination. *Bull. Hist. Med.* 55: 17–33. 1981.

Estes, J. W. Naval medicine in the age of sail: the voyage of the *New York, 1802–1803, Bull. Hist. Med.* 56: 238, 253. 1982.

Goodyear, J. D. The sugar connection: a new perspective on the history of yellow fever. *Bull. Hist. Med.* 52: 5–21. 1978.

Janssens, U. Matthieu Maty and the adoption of inoculation for smallpox in Holland. *Bull. Hist. Med.* 55: 246–256. 1981.

Lentz, G. Outfitting the compleat physician's field kit of 1803. *We Proceeded On* 26: 10–17. 2000.

Niebyl, P. H. The English bloodletting revolution, or modern medicine before 1850. *Bull. Hist. Med.* 51: 464–483. 1977.

Norris, J. The "scurvy disposition": heavy exertion as an exacerbating influence on scurvy in modern times. *Bull. Hist. Med.* 57: 326–338. 1983.

Risse, G. B. Epidemics and medicine: the influence of disease on medical thought and practice. *Bull. Hist. Med.* 53: 505–519. 1979.

Shryock, R. H. The medical reputation of Benjamin Rush: contrasts over two centuries. *Bull. Hist. Med.* 45: 507–552. 1971.

Will, D. The medical and surgical practice of the Lewis and Clark expedition. *J. Hist. Med.* 14: 273–297. 1959.

Index